May Yue's

Tao of Youth™

May Yue's

Tao of Youth™

Let nature heal you

May K. Y. Yue

and

Samuel Ka-Sheng Yue, M.D.

with

Ellen B. Green

Minneapolis • Tao of Youth Publishing • 2007

© 2007 by Tao of Youth Publishing
A division of SKY BioHealth Solutions, Inc.
10300 Valley View Road
Eden Prairie, Minnesota 55344
952-946-1550
Toll-free 888-946-1622
Website: www.taoofyouth.com

ISBN-13: 978-0-9794923-0-3
ISBN-10: 0-9794923-0-0
Library of Congress Control Number: 2007902142

Printed in Hong Kong

10 9 8 7 6 5 4 3 2 1

Cover background image: Jacque Rosenau & Gary Hovda
Cover and text design: Margaret Chan
Editing, layout, production: E. B. Green Editorial, St. Paul, Minnesota
Indexing: Patricia Green, Homer, Alaska

Contents

Key 4
Understanding the Whole You: Unifying Mind, Body, and Spirit

Key 5
Understanding Your Largest Organ: Skincare from the Inside Out

Acknowledgments

Sam and I believe the birthing of this book has followed the law of the universe and that from its conception it has been and is an organic combustion of the energies of people and their ideas. We are grateful for being able to tap into the knowledge of the universe.

Beyond our universal gratitude, we take this opportunity to thank the people who in some fashion directly strengthened this work, whether by giving encouragement when we needed it most, suggesting a special healing soup, or helping to design our cover.

Special thanks to Ellen Green for helping Sam and me put this book together. Without her we would not been able to do it so well. Grateful thanks to Gary Hovda for letting us use his music; it inspired our concept of the *Tao of Youth*. And to our sister Cathy for keeping up to date on health newsletter tips and for supporting our pursuit of the *Tao of Youth*. To Margaret Chan for the beautiful book cover and to Jacque Rosenau for hours spent creating the cover background.

Thanks also to the following persons who assisted us in many different ways: Heidi Chung, Katie Anderson, Susan Mundale, Barbara Forster, Anne Nicolai, Laiki Huxorli, Herb Kearse, Rusty and Eddy Robertson, Esperanza Guerrero, Christine Wai-Werner, Rosa Wong, Yin Simpson, Anne Walcott Sween, Loren Daniels, Louisa Eng, Maria M. Malooly, and Margaret Chan.

Finally we thank all those who have attended our workshops and so refined this work.

Introduction

Overview

I believe that—at any age—to feel my best on the inside and look my best on the outside is healthy. The effects of looking good and feeling good are mutual—they work together, each enhancing the other. I also believe that using nature/science and personal effort together will accomplish both.

Don't get me wrong—I don't oppose plastic surgery or other outside help to make anyone feel beautiful. Gravity does take over, however, and no matter how much you work to stop it, one day you will look and feel older. But why not use what we have discovered to feel and look your best at whatever age you are? And why not use it to feel and look your best as you recover from surgery? In fact, it will help you to recover!

May Yue's Tao of Youth: Let Nature Heal You advocates a five-step process for cleansing the body of toxins and physically turning back time. It works for everyone.

Based on hundreds of published studies in both Eastern and Western medicine plus ten years of research and discovery by my brother Sam Yue, M.D., the *Tao of*

Youth works from the inside out—to reverse the effects of toxins and generate the feeling and appearance of youth. The steps are simple:

1. Understanding Water Gain versus Fat Gain
2. Understanding Your Internal Fountain of Youth
3. Understanding Posture: What Are You Doing at the Gym?
4. Understanding the Whole You: Unifying Mind, Body, and Spirit
5. Understanding Your Largest Organ: Skincare from the Inside Out.

The *Tao of Youth* works *with* the body's natural desires and tendencies, not against them. It's easier than dieting—no deprivation or uncomfortable routine. It's based on science and age-old, proven realities of graceful aging—an art perfected by my great-grandmother, who lived well to the age of 105.

Everybody's heard you must retire at age 65, move south to a warmer climate, enjoy a life of leisure, behave in a certain way. The body aches, the mind fogs, and the spirit fades. That's how it is. You must accept it. But must you really?

We set out to learn how some people, especially those living in Asian countries, have been able to lead vibrant lives to a ripe old age. We have met with hundreds of people in dozens of focus groups and medical workshops in several countries. My brother, Dr. Sam Yue, has treated thousands in his pain clinic, where many of our remedies came to light. Those who have heard about and used our suggestions clamor for more—for something in writing, something to take home, some way to share with others. Thus, this volume. Here's how our approach differs from others:

1. Conventional wisdom is often mistaken. We try to understand the convention-al idea, then look beyond its face to the hidden questions. Through intuitive deduction, we often come up with an answer that works.
2. Experts often use or share information to serve a certain agenda. We do our own research, find information, compare, and learn. We try to understand the origins of the answers of the experts. Then we "sleuth" with no agenda, incen-

tive (such as the promise of a research grant), or self-interest other than to find out what will keep us healthy and young. We have put that together with medical knowledge and day-to-day experience with patients and others to find an alternative course.

3. We approach problems in everyday living from the perspective of Chinese Americans with knowledge of both Chinese traditional and Western medicine.

Curiosity makes the difference. The curious physician continues to learn, to question conventional wisdom, to give the best of care. My brother is one of these. He asks many questions; so do I. Here are some questions prompting our research:

- Why do most female chronic-pain patients suffer less during pregnancy?
- Why do we hear about only two female hormones, when actually there are three?
- Why do women gain weight around their middles after a certain age?
- Metabolism decreases with age. But are there other reasons for weight gain?
- Why does no amount of weightlifting rid me of bouncy flesh around my arms and neck?
- How can women achieve younger figures without starving themselves?
- Why are there more overweight people in northern than in southern China?
- Why do women end up with osteoporosis even when they eat foods loaded with calcium?
- Why do women age so suddenly after menopause? What can they do about it?
- Why do pregnant women have such a glow? How can others have it too?
- Why isn't camellia-seed oil, which is loaded with oleic acid considered good for skincare, not available in the United States?
- Is there any way to arrive at nirvana without chanting for two hours before dawn?

I began asking these questions in my forties; my brother has helped me to answer them. As a younger woman, I wondered, "What kind of older woman am I becoming?" Now the question I have asked for a long time is more important: "What are the fundamentals of aging well?" The answers I have found are contained here.

We know there are many health-and-wellness books addressing the concept of aging well. But the *Tao of Youth* is unique in presenting concepts and findings that make common sense but may be controversial because, inexplicably, no popular books on health and wellness have presented them. Neither has the medical community recognized all of our ideas.

Not that all the concepts are new—though some are presented in new ways, asking questions that most experts have not. We don't presume to know everything about any topic, so we have asked experts in healthcare and other fields for answers. As a result, we present findings old and new and provide a fresh way of looking at them both.

We often present information as a series of questions and answers, in which I represent the everyday aging person, asking questions of my brother Sam, a physician. He bypasses medical jargon and explains things in ways easy for the layperson to understand. We use simple words in offering the five keys to the *Tao of Youth*.

We present here what we have learned in our own aging processes and during years of work with thousands of patients in Sam's pain clinics. We see the need for additional research in some areas—our presentation might be thought of as a white paper in recognizing that need.

So I have written this volume with my brother Dr. Sam Yue's help to provide healthy guidelines for aging to the ordinary reader. For the past ten years we have carried on research, interviewed experts, and used the suggested steps ourselves and with other members of our family. My brother's observations of good results in patients and others attending our workshops have prompted us to share the *Tao of Youth* with a larger sphere.

We choose to empower our readers rather than tell them what to do. We want you to be the master of your own mind, body, and spirit. We do not mean for you to become an expert but for you to become more aware of the right questions, so that you and your healthcare provider can make the best choices for you. We are not here to advise you in a health crisis. Instead, we focus on promoting health and redefining the process of aging so that you live actively, productively, and joyfully.

Furthermore, we present you with a set of new assumptions about aging, because we know that if you understand the fundamentals and ask the right questions, you will be able to make the best healthcare decisions.

For example on another front, I have been able to master the skill of cooking because as part of my major in college, I studied the principles of cooking—with an emphasis on biochemistry. Like the *Iron Chef* of cable television fame (I am not as good as that but good enough to perform in my own kitchen), I am able to come up with something to make from any ingredient, usually without a recipe. I know the rules, so I can mix and match. In the same way, I learned business principles and disciplines. I used those principles in running a software company, and now I use them in managing a biotech and wellness firm. I don't need different principles for each.

With the same kind of thinking, I have come to see a need for new principles and assumptions regarding aging, beauty, and health. Enough to ask, in every instance, "What are the right and crucial questions?" Why new assumptions? Because we live in a time of new realities.

When members of my class asked my favorite marketing professor, Marty Marshall, for notes on how he arrived at a particular set of assumptions, he said, "I won't hand out these notes because I want you to understand that reality is affected by economic, political, and historical change. My job is to give you the skills to figure it out, not to spoonfeed you."

I have never forgotten Professor Marshall's lecture. In the same way, I hope you will read for an understanding of mind and body so that you can comfortably make decisions to improve your health—before it is in crisis.

My brother and I set out to understand how we age and what we can do about it because we and other members of our family are going through middle life. In addition to our research and its application to ourselves, to Sam's patients, and to those of his fellow physicians, Sam and I for seven years have worked as partners to formulate and market products based on his patents and inventions. In that work I have met many experts at conferences and consumers at workshops we have led.

Throughout this volume you will find the sets of assumptions leading to our conclusions: we know that in some areas more research is needed. Some findings may be controversial. We have done our best. We speak our truth. We share this information so that you can, if you choose, lead a better and healthier life.

Background

Our family's story is similar to that of other immigrants. Four generations migrated three times, until we settled in the United States.

Our great-grandmother, Ah Ma, left her opium-addicted husband because he was ready to sell her to satisfy his habit. The bound-footed Ah Ma moved south with her five-year-old son (our grandfather) from Nanda to the town of Putian in Fujian, China. She worked as a maid for a missionary couple, and her son apprenticed for the husband, who was a certified Royal British Surgeon.

Later our grandfather became a certified surgeon too. He started a medical school and eventually owned much land and many businesses. He raised six children—four sons and a daughter who became physicians, and another daughter, who earned a doctorate at Johns Hopkins University in the early 1920s. As superintendent of the major Hong Kong hospitals, our father (the third son) helped bring the system to a modern standard of care. All his sons (my brothers), including Sam, are physicians too.

We grew up in Taipo Market (a fishing village outside Hong Kong), where we moved to escape Communism. We lost everything and had to start again—in fact, we had to borrow boat fare from our tailor to go from Putian to Hong Kong. We lived in Taipo Market from the time I was four years old until I was 14, then settled in nearby Kowloon. Both Sam and I came to the United States for college.

A particular photograph hanging on a wall in our parents' home fascinated me as a child. It showed Ah Ma's (my great-grandmother's) 100th-birthday party with members of four generations surrounding her. She was the oldest in the photo. I was the youngest, and I sat on Ah Ma's lap.

To me that photo represents the spirit of the Yue family. Some members have since passed away, yet because of Ah Ma's bravery, the essence and values of the family passed forward to this generation and will go on to the next. The photo I gazed on long ago now hangs in a special place in my home.

So, our family has a long-life history. Ah Ma thrived until she was 105 and died of natural causes. She went through life-changing moves and political changes in China. Her life was not easy, yet she was alert until the day she died. Since Ah Ma's death, our family has continued her story of change and adaptation, though now all are settled in the Twin Cities (St. Paul and Minneapolis), Minnesota, USA.

Because of this story and through the example of members of our family, we have developed drives and perspectives different from most others we have known. Our values are different—we do not take things for granted, for instance, because we do not know when we may move again. Neither are we attached to things—we literally dropped everything and started over, and we may have to do it again.

There is a Chinese saying: "We start our lives with our bare hands." This can-do attitude is reminiscent of the mindset and entrepreneurial spirit of the American frontier. We learned early to rely on ourselves. The only constancy is change: everything else is in flux.

Ah Ma (a child bride) showed great courage in leaving her household and starting a new life. Our parents' escape to Hong Kong was also a brave act. Our father went first, and our mother followed a year later, with six children (ages 2 to 9), on the last ferry.

These real-life stories showed us the value of making difficult choices for the better. We must face difficult situations with courage. One hesitation could turn us (and others) from a right to a wrong direction. More important, the stories taught us to follow our inner voices, to serve the needs of others in choosing a profession. The generations before us used these principles to create and improve their lives and the lives of those around them.

Sam and I were born in Fujian, China, in a family with six children. He is number three and I number four in sibling order. We worked together briefly in a business we owned together before Sam decided to go back to medical school. He graduated from the University of the East Ramon Magsaysay Medical Center, in the Philippines, as a pain specialist and now has a successful practice in St. Paul.

Meanwhile, I moved into the finance/investment world. On a fellowship I completed OPM work at the Harvard Business School, then for six years ran a software company for Bill Norris after he retired from Control Data. Seven years ago, Sam and I went into partnership to form SKY BioHealth Solutions, Inc., which sells products based on Sam's inventions and patents. We enjoy working together again.

As children—just a year apart in age, with similar approaches to life and little disagreement—we were close. As adults, we complement each other in our strengths and compensate for each other's weakness. Each of us constantly challenges the other's thinking. We are curious and love to learn, and we are open to new ideas. We help each other when times are tough. We are soul mates as well as siblings.

Once when I was in kindergarten, Sam (in a different grade) took part in a school play. Sam played the king, and I was the princess. On the stage, I said my lines, then waited for the king's royal entrance. I waited and waited until I heard my teacher say from backstage: "Follow my words and sing." The song was not part of the script, but I followed, line by line and verse by verse. Finally Sam entered, crying because his beard hurt his chin. The audience laughed and clapped. In the end it was a good experience. You see we have been collaborating for a long time.

East Meets West

While reading many English and Chinese books about health and wellness, to prepare for writing this volume, I was struck by how young Western medicine is in comparison to that of the ancient Chinese.

My own grandfather, Zhin Tao Yue, was the first to introduce Western medicine to the part of China where I was born. He died before I grew up, but my father told me he first brought Western health practices to the villagers of the Putian, Fujian, area. A certified Royal British Surgeon, he evacuated many villages because the residents were dying of a plague spread by rats carrying germs due to bad sanitation. He used disinfectants to stop the spread of disease, a practice learned from a missionary, and introduced Western surgery there. Though his methods might today seem primitive, he was advanced for his day, and he saved many lives.

Grandfather—a healer not prejudiced about whom he would treat—was the most influential person in his area. When a wealthy person's son was kidnapped, he asked my grandfather to negotiate the ransom. He was the only one trusted to go blindfolded to where the bandits lived and to get the job done. My mother, at age 91 the oral historian of our family, says he was an intuitive healer—sometimes he looked at a patient across the room and just knew what was wrong. He was a "karma doctor."

When in World War II the Chinese government combined many regional schools of medicine to form the Beijing Medical School, Grandfather merged his own medical school with that one. Today it is one of the most prestigious in China. Still, he had no problem using old remedies along with antibiotics and surgery. One prized remedy was a jar of decomposing tangerine peels he used to treat patients with boils. The faint scar on my forehead, I am told, is from a boil treated in that way.

The Western medicine that took hold during my grandfather's era evolved into the most powerful way of delivering medicine to the masses; its influence was worldwide and trumped most forms of traditional medicine. My family benefited from the trend. My oldest uncle was the first Chinese surgeon to graduate from a school in England; he was the medical director for all the clinics and hospitals in Southeast Asia for the Church of England. At age 28 my father, Man Young Yue, was asked to run St. Luke's Hospital in Fujian.

When we left China to escape Communism, my father knew his experience as a hospital administrator would be valued in Hong Kong. He worked 30 years (from the 1950s to the 1980s) as superintendent of the major government hospitals there, bringing them into the 20th century. Queen Elizabteth, Queen Mary, and the Tong Wah Group Hospitals, with 2,000 to 3,000 beds each, served 6.5 million citizens.

Father's last major assignment was with Caritas Hospital (a Catholic branch from Germany), which he transformed into a thriving entity serving the poor.

In this generation, my brother, Dr. Sam Yue, noticed that what he learned in Western medical schools was not enough. So he started learning on his own, and through 20 years of medical practice, he has combined Eastern with Western approaches to medicine.

My grandfather, my father, his brothers, and my brother have been gifted, compassionate "karma doctors." All used both Western technology and ancient wisdom. This approach is just what we need in today's wellness revolution—a vast increase in expectations for wellness as we age. With our unique heritage—as products of both East and West—Sam and I offer you the best of what we know of both worlds.

I have discovered in my quest for wellness that combining Western and Eastern ways is the best path. Traditional Chinese Medicine brings so much ancient wisdom to the table—yet I would not dream of going without the Western testing, for example, that monitors my progress. Nor would I eschew the hospital or a good Western physician for surgery. This integrated approach, attuned to the philosophy of the Tao, is my way—using what I see as best, wherever I find it, to follow my path.

So all our research and reading of the experts comes to this: For harmony and balance of the life force, for the best health and continued wellness as we age, we must first pay attention to the health of our

- cells (building blocks of the body)
- circulation (blood flow and blood vessels)
- glands (for hormone balance)

We can do that best by eating foods that keep cells, blood vessels, and glands and glandular production in good order. When food is not enough, food supplements can be a strategy for extra advantage. With cellular, circulatory, and glandular health in order (because all other systems depend on them), whatever we can do for the following systems will increase wellness and longevity:

- digestive system
- lymphatic system
- all organs
- bones
- muscles

We use both Eastern and Western practices. We eat what is healthy, sometimes looking to foods prescribed by ancient wisdom. We use modern tests for establishing baselines, developing plans for improvement, monitoring progress. We exercise for muscle and bone health, work to achieve serenity, sometimes using modern technology and sometimes using effective, ancient practices to maintain wellness for as long as we can.

How will the *Tao of Youth* help you achieve these objectives?

- Key 1 addresses eating the right kinds of foods and the flushing of toxins and water weight towards cellular and artery health, towards healthy digestive and lymphatic systems.
- Key 2 addresses hormone balance, little understood by most people, including those in the medical profession. For optimum health and a tremendous edge in the battle to age well, learn as much about this topic as you can and follow through with what is best for you.
- Key 3, with the backup of my brother's experience as a physician treating patients with chronic pain, addresses posture—or more specifically, muscle and bone health.
- Key 4 addresses the integration of body, mind, and spirit, showing how music of a certain frequency can reduce stress and help you stay in an alpha (calm and high-functioning) state.
- Key 5 addresses the state of your skin—the largest organ, the one most reflecting the state of your health. Topical creams may help, but for beautiful skin you must be well in body, mind, and spirit.

The goal is to reestablish the life force providing the ultimate gift—life lived as you know and dream it can be. When your body works harmoniously, when it is healthy, there is an equilibrium in which lie connection, harmony, balance—a resonance of mind, body, and spirit. When these are not in sync, when you are "out of tune," there is only chaos—and possibly serious disease.

Chaos hits everyone now and then—it is like a forest fire. You must act quickly to put out the flames. No one option is the answer; you muster your power and focus to take charge, to engage the best offensive strategy. Your physician may help you put out the fire, but he or she is not the chief of your fire department. You must engage in the effort to achieve your "state of enviable health." You are the chief of your personal health department. Take charge.

What Is Tao?

Tao is the ultimate principle binding all existence together. Existence is a vast playful dance, a cosmos of great order. The name of that order is *Tao*, the harmony of the whole. The closest English word for Tao is *Nature*.

Tao is spontaneity—a state of letting go. Tao is not about doing—not about developing character, discipline, or even conscience—but about being, in tune with existence. There is no separation. You are not the wave but the sea. Be what you are—just yourself—here and now. Be conscious of every part. Accept who you are. Allow your inner contradictions to fall in love so that the conflicts disappear. Declare you uniqueness. Surrender your ego. You are man and woman, east and west, science and meditation. The earth is one village. Be one with the dance of the world.

Be simple and spontaneous. Put fear aside. Let go. Open your heart. See with a fresh eye. Be free, and your fears disappear. Drown yourself in the bounty of the world, in all its colors. Laugh, love, and celebrate totally, without seeking permanence. The beauty of life is that it is always a surprise. Accept life totally, and every moment becomes juicy—nirvana. Celebrate the gift of life—the only true prayer.

Tao flourishes in this moment. Live it in purity and silence, spontaneity and gratitude. You need not push the river. You simply allow it to take you to the sea.

Characteristics of Those Who Follow the Tao

1. Sensitivity: Those who follow the Tao are observant of others, avoid aggression, and help others in need. They love nature and study the creativity of nature. Through nature, they glimpse the Tao.
2. Independence: They do not focus on fads, trends, or political movements, which are too confining. They value wisdom and experience far over government or conventional behavior and etiquette.
3. Flexibility: They rarely rule anything out because they believe any choice they make depends on circumstances rather than on preconceived notions.
4. Focus: They learn an inner direction in their lives. They accept who they are. They do not try to be someone they are not. They take advantage of their best attributes and set out to work with them as best they can.
5. Discipline: They take orderly actions towards a specific goal; this requires concentration of the highest order.
6. Compassion: They seek a sense of wholeness through nature and spontaneity. Compassion is their impulse towards others. "Every act has Good and Evil results." The natural and spontaneous people will always choose the good—the path allowing the natural flow of life to guide their actions.
7. Joy: They feel directly connected to the source of life. They do not fear poverty because they feel rich. They do not feel loneliness because they are their own good companions. They do not fear death because their experience remains no matter what else happens—the soul lives on. They live in nirvana.

How to Apply the Tao

The study of Tao originated in China thousands of years ago. Since Tao is the total ongoing process of the universe, it makes sense to follow it rather than to go against it. Tao is a way of life guiding you to rich experience. It is a spiritual path of joy, insight, and freedom.

Those interested in Tao usually begin by reading *Tao Tse Ching,* written by Taoist sage Lao Tze of the Zhou dynasty, about 2,600 years ago. From there, they often go to *I Ching*, which gives insight into the cosmological concepts of Taoism and uses chance as a mean of connecting with Tao for the purpose of divination. There are Tao-related volumes of history, novels, and poetry, as well as works on herbal medicine, acupuncture, art, martial arts, longevity, exercise, ritual, and even sorcery.

But what do the ramblings of sages 2,000 years ago have to do with me?

We must go on with our lives now, facing what comes our way. We may think of Tao while we are working. We may wonder what the sages would say while we are trying to make sense of our lives. Little has been written on how to apply Tao to modern life. How do we apply the wisdom of ancient masters to what we face now?

If we truly understand Tao, we don't need endless theory. Tao shows us a person on a path—one who may represent all of humanity or even the universe. The path contains movement, balance, and harmony. Once we begin a journey on the path, all the teachings of Tao open to us. The ultimate learning of Tao is not the accumulation of book knowledge but the application of our understandings to daily life. The *Tao of Youth* is a pursuit of everyday wellness based on the wisdom of the Tao.

As described earlier, this book is divided into five keys, or steps on a path—the *Tao of Youth*—to feeling healthy and young. Like the five fingers of a hand, the sections seem separate. They look different from one another, and they have separate functions. Yet also like fingers of a hand, together they work as a whole.

You probably have injured a finger and found your routine disrupted when you couldn't use it with the others. This is the case with body, mind, spirit. You represent a part of nature—all your inner workings are a part of nature. With natural movement, balance, and harmony, you are at your best and enjoy life the most. Finding the balance upon which traditional Chinese medicine is based will ease your path.

In terms of the Tao, Keys 1 and 2 to the *Tao of Youth* deal with the inner workings of your physical body—how we have used Tao and how you can use it to understand your system in ways beyond those of the Western world, beyond giving away your personal power to the "experts."

How do we combine understanding, common sense, and knowledge from both East and West to regain the natural flow of movement and achieve optimum health? Just as nature inspired the ancients to follow Tao, so we understand Tao through the world around us. To follow the path, we realize we are a part of nature.

The reality is that for the sake of "progress" we sometimes forget Tao—the forgetting gets us into trouble in our everyday lives. The trick is to discover how to live with the progress of civilization and still be in balance with the universe. So in Keys 1 and 2, we show you how we arrived and how you can arrive at the best strategies to keep your body in working order, just as nature intended.

In Key 3, we deal with the pragmatic side of Tao's teaching, taking a look at the outside physical appearance of the body, asking how we can become well-informed, then learning and applying our knowledge so that we can feel and look our best.

Tao accepts, with other Asian spiritual systems such as Buddhism and Hinduism, that material reality is ultimately an empty illusion. Still, the ancients recognized that most of the time we cannot function in a state of realized emptiness. We live in the real world. Everyday life lived to advantage ultimately provides the basis for a spiritual life.

With Key 4 we develop the spiritual aspect of Tao. The abundant self-help books of the day indicate that many members of our generation seek enlightenment. We also realize that you must deal with the physiological—thus our discussion of the lymphatic system. No amount of psychotherapy or prayer will supply nutrients to your brain or balance your bodily systems. But on the path of Tao, we accept the tools and remedies available and ask, "What is the best strategy?" We take into account the idea of change set forth in *I Ching* (see Appendix) as well as the art of strategy treated in Sunzi's *Art of War.*

Life changes and progresses in cycles documented by the ancients. Following Tao enables us to apply these principles directly to life. Tao helps us to avoid excess and frustration though a gradual looking into the self and ultimately takes us to self-realization. We then live wiser lives.

Key 5 returns to the pragmatic. Tao is unique in asserting that the everyday reality experienced on the way to a higher spiritual life is worth pursuing. Tao does not teach that you must be a hermit or live on the mountain, away from the outside world. Caring for your largest organ—your skin—reflects your way of life. Your skin plays a big part of your first impression on others. Problems with your skin show that you may be straying from the Tao. We use Tao to pursue understanding and provide the best strategies to achieve healthy and beautiful skin.

Like the fingers of your hand, the five keys seem unrelated, look different, and function separately, yet they are interrelated parts of the *Tao of Youth* system of wellness. Use the *Tao of Youth* from the inside out. Be a part of nature, part of the order of the cosmos, and live the Tao of joy and happiness. Whatever and wherever you are on your path is valid. Inquiry and action begin with you.

Key 1

Understanding water gain versus fat gain

What We Saw

Growing older is not so tough after all! As I watched my mother age, I thought that I would be in for a hard time. But in fact I feel a lot better about myself now than when I was younger. Freedom comes with age—you let go of a lot and don't take things so seriously. I enjoy life.

But I really dislike one aspect of aging—that roll around my middle.

Before reaching menopause, I could eat anything I wanted and still weigh the same. I was a size six for decades. Then, in my early fifties, I suddenly noticed I had two bellies—one above the naval and another below. I no longer had a waist—I looked like a watermelon!

I tried on my pants and T-shirts, horrified at the sight in the mirror, unable to tuck in a shirt and still fasten my pants. I ran out to a department store for some new clothes, ending up with several Eileen Fisher ensembles—of beautiful fabrics and straight, roomy lines.

I noticed that other women my age were dressing the same way, but I still wanted the size-six me. What was happening to us? Could I change it? I began to ask a lot of questions.

I also tried many diets, none of which seemed to work for me. Well, some worked for awhile, but I always gained back the weight—and the diets did not fit my daily lifestyle. Maybe I would just have to live with the extra weight—like other women my age.

Meanwhile my niece, Lindsey (Sam's daughter), age 16, was studying abroad, in Beijing, China. She weighed 125 pounds when she left but 165 pounds upon her return a year later. She had ballooned like me!

During her stay in Beijing, Lindsey lived with a family that served and ate noodles, dumplings, and steamed buns every day, as do most of the people in northern China. Lindsey and I were not the same age, but we had the same problem!

During a visit to Hong Kong that year, I asked a doctor of traditional Chinese medicine (TCM) to take a pulse reading to see what was wrong with my body. He did and said, "You have a Dampness and Heat problem." This meant my body contained too much water and that I was overnourished—as opposed to having a Dry and Cold condition (being without water and undernourished). He wrote me a prescription for an herbal remedy.

I asked my brother Sam a lot of questions about my niece's weight gain and my own problem with extra weight. I discovered that Sam and I are both curious people, and that when we encounter a mystery, we work well as partners in solving it. For lack of a better term, I have come to call what we do "sleuthing." In this search, particularly, Sam showed discipline in asking the theoretical questions, and I kept him honest by asking the practical questions pertinent to everyday life.

Sam told me, for instance, that Lindsey's weight gain did not make sense in calorie theory. At her rate of calorie intake, it would have taken her two to three years to gain as much weight as she did.

During surgeries, Sam had noticed that a lot of water leaked from the body tissues of female and overweight male patients. He was puzzled by the phenomenon and asked other surgeons whether they had noticed the same thing. They said, yes, they had noticed water in the area between tissues. Most of them just left it at that, but Sam kept reading and wondering about the cause of the leaking.

Then Sam noticed something in examining patients for the diagnosis of fibromyalgia—recognized as positive if there has been pain for at least three months and pain at more than 11 of 18 pressure-point sites. He found the tissue around the lymphatic areas of these patients especially puffy.

Hmmm . . . the bulkiness in my aging body weight concentrated in my midsection, shoulders, and neck area—all close to the lymph nodes.

Searching for answers, Sam looked up the herbs prescribed for me by the doctor in China. Then I found the famous Li Shi-zhen's herbal medicine book *Ben Cao Gang Mu* or *The Great Pharmacopoeia*. In this book, Sam found a list of the same herbs prescribed for releasing dampness some 400 years ago. Though they cannot explain why the herbs "release dampness," the Chinese have known their effect for hundreds of years.

Sam made another observation when we were traveling to meetings in China. In the north the diet is mostly wheat, while in the south, where we grew up, the people eat rice and rice noodles. And there is a definite difference in the general weight of people living south and north. Those in the north are much heavier.

Back in the United States, Sam asked a few of his patients to replace the wheat and dairy products in their diets with rice and potatoes for two months. They came back 20 to 30 pounds lighter. This was another puzzle—under the theory of calorie intake, you could never lose that much weight in such a short time! Sam set out to solve it.

What Sam found now helps me, my niece, and many of his patients control weight and feel better—not through a strategy of dieting but by being in charge of our own bodies, by replenishing them with nutrients that help our systems to work better.

My niece and I have something in common—a weak digestive system. She inherited hers, and mine has become less effective with age. But I am happy to say that after learning how to eat in a healthy way, we have lost weight and improved our immune systems as well as our general health.

Our approach may seem strange. The experts argue that calorie intake is the most important element in weight loss and gain. But they have overlooked what is right before our eyes. The truth is that we must pay attention to the water in our bodies as well as to calorie intake and exercise. But most people in the United States are not tuned to their bodies or to their reactions to certain foods.

Finding out how to change my eating habits to achieve and maintain a healthy weight as I age has demanded experimentation—trial and error. The approach we take makes the journey a work in progress, but I have found some things that work and wish to share them here.

But first, Sam's explanation of water vs. fat weight—or how to put your digestive and lymphatic systems in good working order.

What We Asked

What's the difference between water weight and fat weight?

You may think a pound is a pound, but there are two kinds of weight gain and the difference is crucial. Excess weight may be categorized as net "fat" weight or as water weight trapped in the lymphatic system (we'll explain that later).

Net fat weight is the result of excessive calorie intake—of simply eating too much, that is, more calories than you burn.

Water weight is the accumulation of water in the lymphatic system—caused by eating certain things that are harder to digest—especially as you get older. The water accompanying partially digested proteins eventually leaks into the lymphatic system, is trapped in the lymph nodes, and blocks the flow of lymph (lymphatic fluids). This results in fluid retention in the lymphatic system. Medical professionals commonly call this condition high-protein edema.

To lose weight, you must differentiate net fat weight from water weight and treat each with appropriate methods.

What role does my digestive system play in water-weight gain?

Certain foods are more difficult to digest than others. All proteins, for instance, are digested into the smallest components—amino acids. These amino acids are absorbed through the linings of the gastrointestinal (GI) tract into the blood. Your body uses amino acids to build various tissues.

As you age, your digestive enzymes diminish, and your body is not able to digest food so thoroughly as when you were younger. Partially digested food (macronutrients consisting of clumps of amino acids) clings to the lining of the GI tract, often leaking into the vascular circulation, or blood. The lining of the intestines and colon (gastrointestinal mucosa) filters out most of the larger undigested macronutrients. But the smaller macronutrients pass through the lining in a condition commonly referred to as Leaky Gut Syndrome (altered permeability of the GI tract). Medical and weight-loss professionals often overlook this condition common to both women and men. Genetics, age, hormones, medications (prednisone, especially), infections, parasites, toxins produced by bacteria or fungi, and many other factors contribute to an increase in the permeability, or leakage, of macronutrients into your blood.

What happens to the undigested proteins that seep into my blood?

While many nutritionists and physicians are familiar with Leaky Gut Syndrome, they assume that the liver detoxifies undigested proteins in the blood. Instead, the lymphatic system provides the disposal system for these clumps of amino acids.

While the liver detoxifies some of the clumps of amino acids delivered from the bloodstream, partially digested protein leaks from the capillaries (the smallest blood vessels) into the interstitial space, or space between the cell walls of your body. Undigested protein (small clumps of amino acids) then drain slowly into your lymphatic system. (See Key 5 for the parts of the overall digestive system.)

What is the lymphatic system and what is it for?

Lymph originates as blood plasma that leaks from the circulatory system into the surrounding tissues. The tissues collect this fluid (lymph) and return it to the circulation while working with your white blood cells to protect your body from infection. There is no central pump, and the movement is slow.

Undigested proteins draining into the lymphatic system may cause extra water retention within the system. Once in, they clump onto the lymph nodes along the entire system. Whenever and wherever clumps of amino acids (foreign proteins, at this point called antigens) drain into the lymph nodes, your body mounts an anti-body or immunity reaction. These form an antigen-antibody complex that blocks drainage from the nodes and lymphatic vessels that drain through them. This slows the drainage of lymph downstream from the interstitial space. The space between the cell walls then swells with water, the basis of high-protein edema.

The extra protein load within the lymph nodes and lymph vessels also draws water into the lymphatic system to balance the osmotic pressure (difference between the amount of protein in the lymphatic fluid and in the blood vessel). The result is an accumulation of water in the lymphatic system and in the interstitial space. This is the water weight that makes many middle-aged persons heavier in their midsections. The heightened immune response, sometimes misdirected to other parts of the body, results in inflammation of those areas too.

What happens then? Why doesn't my lymphatic system take care of it?

Once the undigested proteins or antigens form antigen-antibody complexes in the lymph nodes, your body begins the slow process of breaking the protein com-plexes into smaller pieces that can drain easily through the lymph nodes, into the larger lymphatic system, and eventually into your bloodstream.

Is there anything I can do to help it?

Clearing and cleaning your lymphatic system, particularly the lymph nodes, al-lows more efficient flow of the lymph. When you flush your lymph nodes clean, you eliminate stored-up, stagnant, lymphatic water—and you get rid of the water weight! This is one of the first things you notice when you go on a high-protein diet—you lose a large amount of weight in the first few weeks. But reduced calorie intake and balance can't alone account for the large weight loss. Even if you consumed no calories during the first month, you could not lose that much "fat." The majority of weight lost in the first few weeks is water. And it is mostly the excessive lymphatic water of high-protein edema.

This probably also accounts for the high and quick water accumulation that occurs once you go back on a regular diet—eating the same "fattening" foods that got you into trouble before.

How can I keep my digestive system clean and avoid the retention of water?

There are many foods not easily digested by some individuals, but two proteins from two food groups stand out as the hardest to digest for most people—gluten, in the grain family—wheat, rye, oats, barley, spelt—and casein, in milk and other dairy products. (See pages 28–29 for listings of the sources of gluten and what you might eat instead.)

What is gluten?

Gluten (a protein in grain that gives dough its elasticity) is a known poison for a small group of individuals who have celiac disease. For these people, eating gluten without treatment eventually results in death. But mild cases of gluten allergy are often overlooked. A milder intolerance of gluten can be the beginning of many digestive problems.

What is casein? I thought lactose was the problem.

Most people know that many are allergic to lactose in dairy products. But lactose is not the cause of extra water weight in the lymphatic system. The culprit is casein, or milk protein. Many infants and children diagnosed as allergic to milk (its lactose or casein) grow out of the condition before adulthood. Many adults allergic to milk take lactose enzyme or Lactaid®. But if casein (a protein with a lot of hard-to-digest amino acids) is the cause of water weight, reducing or eliminating lactose will not solve the problem.

But I have eaten wheat and milk products for many years without any problem. What's wrong now?

As you age, your body secretes fewer and fewer of the enzymes necessary to digest many of the things you ate without weight gain when you were younger. Fewer enzymes compound the slowdown of your digestive process and magnify the harmful effects of the two protein groups—gluten and casein. That's why a teenager can polish off a whole pizza alone, but by the time you turn 50, you have trouble digesting a single slice. Pizza, a favorite of many Americans, is—you guessed it—mainly gluten and casein.

So as you get older, it's a good idea to gradually reduce your consumption of—or avoid completely—the two foods that contribute greatly to lymphatic water retention for most people—gluten and casein. For many people, there are other offending foods as well.

Must I cut out all pasta, cereal, bread, every dessert, even ice cream? Is there anything else I can do?

You can supplement digestive enzymes orally to help your body digest and absorb nutrients and avoid partially digested protein. Whenever you eat offending foods, use digestive enzymes to help the digestive process.

What are these enzymes? What are they made of?

There are two basic types of digestive enzymes—plant-based and animal-based.

Plant-based enzymes, such as papain from papaya, help you to digest protein almost immediately after ingesting the offending food. This is the enzyme you buy at the grocery store to tenderize meat.

Animal-based enzymes work best when your body pH (the ratio of acidity to alkalinity within your body—a pH of 7 is neutral, below 7 is acidic, and above 7 is alkaline) is more alkaline. Animal-based enzymes are similar to those secreted by your pancreas. They break protein, fat, and carbohydrates into simpler components so that your blood can more easily absorb them.

A full digestive process, enhanced by supplemental digestive enzymes as you age, allows less leakage of undigested protein and less lymphatic accumulation. A combination of plant- and animal-based enzymes works the best.

How can I flush out the water and toxins that are already in my lymphatic system? What foods, herbs, and supplements will help?

Once you eliminate the effect of toxic foods in accumulating lymphatic water, you can take steps to flush the toxins and extra water from your system. Many colon cleansing, purging, and detoxification products are commercially available to clean the intestines and colon, or gut. Using them may help to reduce the undigested proteins in the lining of the gut, but they will not flush out the lymphatic system.

Many physicians prescribe Lasix® (a common diuretic) to patients complaining of generalized swelling, particularly in their lower extremities. Many people have used this diuretic for months, even years, without resolution of the swelling. This is because the lymphatic system, not the blood, retains the water. No amount of diuretic will get rid of it. At most, the diuretic will slightly ease some swelling, but the swelling will return when you stop using the diuretic.

If purging products and diuretics won't work, what will?

There are several ways to flush extra water from the lymphatic system. One of the easiest methods is do it naturally. Many raw fruits and vegetable contain digestive enzymes plus healthy bioflavonoids and antioxidants (substances that provide beneficial effects to your body). *Cooking destroys most of these enzymes!* So eating lots of raw vegetables and fruits will help your body get rid of extra water in your lymphatic system.

But when I eat raw fruits and vegetables I have other digestive problems. What can I do about that?

You can increase your intake of raw fruits and vegetable without worrying about extra fiber—which in some people results in gas, bloating, or excessive bowel movements—by juicing the fruits and vegetables. You can also supplement your diet with freeze-dried fruit and vegetable powder or capsules. Freeze-dried, fermented vegetables, as well as the sprouts of many seeds such as barley grass, are full of enzymes for better digestion and flushing of the lymphatic system.

Herbs such as horse chestnut and supplements containing hesperidin (present in oranges and lemons) and diosmin (a vascular-protecting agent) are used in Europe for flushing the lymphatic system. The decongestant guaifenesin also helps flushing for some people.

What about Eastern medicine?

In traditional Chinese medicine, or TCM, conditions such as Leaky Gut Syndrome, lymphedema, and inflammation are classified under the general category Heat and Dampness. These conditions, mimicking over-nutrition (eating too much), occurred only in the upper and ruling classes of ancient Chinese society.

In modern Chinese societies such as Hong Kong, however, Leaky Gut Syndrome, lymphedema, and inflammation are commonly diagnosed. The Chinese physicians distinguish the water retention or edema of the vascular system from the Heat and Dampness of lymphatic water. They use two classes of herbal medication for treatment.

The treatment of Heat and Dampness calls for herbs and teas that contain enzymes, bioflavonoids, and antioxidants effective in flushing the lymphatic zone.

What are these herbs and teas?

Not all herbs and teas are created equal—Oolong tea, for instance, is notable for its flushing ability. (See page 38 for choosing/brewing tea for best results and pages 139, 153–55 and 158, for herb use. See Resources for where to find them.)

How will I know that the flushing has worked?

During flushing with any of the above, you will probably notice increases in urine volume and frequency and changes in color (a deeper yellow), and odor. This is the result of breakdown of the protein complexes in your lymph system and the shifting of fluid from the lymphatic to the vascular system. After the shift, your kidneys take over, and you eliminate the toxins from your body.

What if my extra weight isn't all water?

After you rid yourself of extra water weight, use a healthy weight-loss system to lose the net fat. Calorie intake (count!), proper portions, types of foods (don't forget to cut the gluten and casein), and proper exercise are important to losing net fat weight and, later, to maintain your ideal weight.

How We Eat Now

So now we know that as we get older our digestive systems do not work as well as they did earlier. What can we do about it?

Since it's all about balancing the system, adding enzymes to help your stomach digest the food you eat makes good sense. So does finding ways to keep the GI tract in tiptop shape (to maintain the integrity of your mucosa). (See page 29 for a list of food supplements that will help your digestive system.)

The next thing is to select foods that do not overload your digestive system. If you continually use an appliance, it breaks down. This can happen in your body, too. The focus of Chinese traditional medicine is the yin-yang effect in the body. An imbalanced digestive system triggers into other systems and can cause problems in those as well.

I have decided not to diet—that is, not to call the way I eat a diet, but rather an eating strategy, the one described here. Of course, you do not have to follow it exactly. Many diet books prescribe to the minute what one must eat, but life is simply not that exact. You may go out with friends or be invited to a cocktail or dinner party or find yourself in many other kinds of eating situations—even at the state fair. You don't need a prescriptive diet but a strategy for eating that will please your taste buds, satisfy your tummy, and keep you young and healthy.

Avoid Difficult-to-digest Foods

Gluten-containing grains

- wheat
- barley
- oats
- rye
- spelt (ancient cousin of wheat, known as faro in Italy and dinkel in Germany)
- Kamut® (ancient cousin of modern durum wheat)

Casein (in all dairy products but butter)

To a lesser extent:

- whey protein
- soy and soy-related foods (10–15 percent of those sensitive to dairy foods have a cross-reaction to soy)
- corn

The most important thing is to know that two food groups become harder to digest as we age. There are some subgroups too. See lists of hard-to-digest foods and easy-to-digest grains above and opposite. My digestive system is in pretty good shape, so I am able to eat foods in those subgroups. Occasionally I even eat foods in the gluten and casein groups. I can do that because I have worked at improving and maintaining the health and balance of my digestive system over several years.

Developing an eating habit that does not include gluten and casein is difficult in the United States because almost 80 percent of the foods prepared here contain items from the gluten and casein (dairy) food groups. For instance, if you go to Starbucks or any other shop for a cup of coffee and decide you want a quick breakfast, what will you pick up? A donut, a muffin, a bagel, or coffee cake! It takes a new mindset to stand back and say, "I'd rather have something else for breakfast." Well, you can still eat your egg and your hash-browns, but cut the toast (even if it's whole wheat).

Enjoy Easy-to-digest, Gluten-free Grains

Rice

Glutinous rice (contains no gluten; it's named so for its stickiness)

*   white, brown, black

Short, medium, and long-grained rice

*   black , red, brown, green, others

Rice- and rice-flour-derived foods

*   rice pasta and noodles, and don't forget rice desserts

Millet (nutlike flavor, filled with protein, fiber, B-complex vitamins including niacin, thiamin, and riboflavin, plus methionine, lecithin, vitamin E, iron, magnesium, phosphorous, and potassium)

Buckwheat

*   cereal (really an herb)
*   flour (for pancakes, bread, muffins, crackers, bagels, cookies, tortillas, etc.)
*   Asian noodles

Others

*   Quinoa (nutritionally a super-grain, really a seed full of potassium, riboflavin plus B vitamins, magnesium, zinc, copper, and manganese, some folate)
*   Amaranth (seed high in protein and fiber plus lysine, methionine, calcium, iron, potassium, phosphorus, and vitamins A and C.
*   Sorghum
*   Teff (ancient cereal grain of minute size, packed with nutrients)
*   Wild rice (highly nutritious grain, not really rice but an annual water-grass seed naturally abundant in cold waters of Minnesota and Canada, a staple of the Ojibwe and Dakota native to the region)
*   Job's tears (Chinese pearl barley, from the corn family, Chinese herb used in the diet therapy of stiff joints, rheumatism, and edema, used alone or in soups)

Just like you, I like all the foods containing gluten and casein. It's not been easy to stop eating them; in fact, I haven't been a true convert until recently. Don't be discouraged; Rome wasn't built in a day. I became a true *Tao of Youth* practitioner only after I found two important bits of information that turned the tide. I share them with you so you can have greater success right away. This is the path—the way of the Tao.

About a year ago, when I was in Hong Kong, I stayed in the lovely residential area of Wanchai, much like Knob Hill in San Francisco. There is an avenue called Star Street—much like Soho, very diverse. You can visit an art gallery or a market in the street. A mixture of locals and expatriates live there.

Strolling down Star Street, I saw a teahouse, recently remodeled, opening for the first time that day. The owner, Leo Kwan, a man with a ponytail, greeted me. Why not enjoy the tea ceremony he offered? I entered and fell in love with the Guangzhou teashop—everything done in such good taste, its owner of interesting character and a tea master with real flair. Leo Kwan told me of his ability to heal people with tea, so I began call him a tea doctor.

I phoned Sam to ask him to join me in the tea shop, to help me find out whether Leo Kwan was for real. They talked for hours, were like soul mates right away. Leo served us a special tea from Phoenix Mountain in Guangzhou. We drank it and immediately noticed a buzz in our heads. He claimed that this tea helped his customers lose a lot of weight. I bought a box to bring back to the United States.

I brewed the tea as Leo taught me and drank it religiously for three months. I noticed that my pants fit better and that the extra rolls around my hips and neck were beginning to disappear. My girlish figure returned. I called Sam—he had not drunk the tea as I had. But when I told him what was happening, he started research to find out why this particular tea made that big a difference.

Sam found that what I was drinking was semi-fermented, high-quality Oolong tea. The legend goes that the tea maker (from Fujian, famous for the tea and the city where Sam and I were born) was carrying baskets of tea leaves to be dried for green tea. On the way, he was so captivated by a stream that he decided to do some fishing there. He let the tea leaves sit in the basket, and they started to ferment—by accident. The tea maker was horrified but decided to dry-roast them anyway. He liked the flavor and began to sell it, with great success. The name he gave the tea—Oolong—means absent-minded accident.

Somehow the semi-fermentation of Oolong draws out the enzymes that break down the proteins caught in the lymphatic system. Oolong tea broke down those extra proteins in my system, and they were eliminated through my kidneys.

I gave my sister some of this tea, she loved it too, and we compared notes. We both noticed that the volume of urine was greater and that its odor was different. We knew it worked. Meanwhile, Dr. Sam was trying out different brands of Oolong. He came to the following conclusions: To be effective for our purposes, the Oolong must be fermented by a reputable teahouse. The process is important—some roast the tea too much—in that case, it has a smoky taste. It must be roasted and fermented to a certain degree, and that is sometimes more costly. (The Chinese spend a lot more money on good tea than we Americans would dream of—$100 a pound or more.)

We tried many brand and kinds, determining that price is not the only factor. The tea must be grown at a high altitude, at least 1,500 meters, or 4,500 feet, above sea level. The severe conditions of the higher altitudes force the tealeaves to produce more antioxidants and riboflavin in order to survive. You get a high grade of Oolong from high altitudes.

I began to recommend to friends and acquaintances that they start a daily tea ritual like mine—even if they had weak GI tracts (some of them cannot drink the juices we suggest until they strengthen their systems) because tea is gentle to the stomach. They saw immediate results—incentive to continue on the path.

Avoid gluten and casein and drink Oolong tea—then what? Once your stomach has stabilized—that is when it feels good and does not act up on you—start the juicing routine described on pages 36–37. The particular fruits called for are the easiest to digest. You can get creative as you get farther into it. I add other fruits too, but I found the combination described there is the most soothing. Drinking the juice and the tea is a great start towards flushing extra water from your lymphatic system.

On a later trip to Hong Kong, I ran into another helpful strategy. This time I stayed in a hotel on Jordan Road between the Tsim Sha Tsui and Mong Kok areas. One morning I was looking for a good breakfast. I found a little place on a side street close to my hotel—it was called Enoch Health Station. The owner, Raymond, introduced me to a physician from Taiwan—Dr. Luke Lin. He helps cancer patients detoxify their bodies by eating the right foods.

Raymond is such a believer in Dr. Lin's detoxification system that he opened this restaurant to introduce the doctor's detox menus. I asked Raymond, "How are you going to stay in business with such a restrictive menu?" He said he was adjusting the menu to cater to the public while maintaining the detoxification principles.

He served me a detoxing breakfast—fruit juice (with all the skin and fiber pulverized), a five-grain rice ball (see pages 39–40), and a steamed sweet potato. I was satisfied the whole day, so I went to the bookstore and bought Dr. Lin's book. I was curious to know whether I could adapt the principles of his detoxifying food program for cancer to everyday living.

What I found was that without bread (or pasta, dumplings, noodles, and so forth), most people do not feel satisfied after a meal. I was not brought up eating bread, but I have lived in the United States longer than in China, and I developed the "bread habit" too. The five-grain rice and a steamed sweet potato definitely satisfy my craving. In his book Dr. Lin notes that if you forget everything else in his system of eating and just eat a sweet potato every day, you will see a difference in your health.

Why not white potatoes? Regular potatoes tend to make the sugar level in your blood (your glycemic index) higher, so that you crave more food. Sweet potatoes don't do that. Now that five-grain rice and sweet potato are part of my daily eating strategy, I am content with the food I eat. (Some beans and grains also have flushing ability. See pages 39–40).

Another help to breaking down proteins in the lymphatic system are the healing soups that the Chinese have enjoyed for centuries. I cannot remember a time when I did not regularly drink soup containing the healing herbs in some way or other. The Chinese people, especially those in southern China, believe soup is a tonic that balances the yin and yang of the body. Hong Kong, for instance, has just opened 20 convenient soup-making shops so that people can order soup and pick it up on their way home from work at the entrances to the subway.

Some families have handed down soup recipes over several generations. I have searched for recipes for healing soups suited to the Western palate that include an explanation of the herbs. Some herbs are more useful for other conditions, some are hard to get, and some are hard to get used to. See pages 41–42 for easy-to-make soups that also tend to break down stray proteins in your lymphatic system.

The Chinese often do not eat the solid part of the soup, ingesting only the liquid as a tonic to soothe the stomach. Give your tummy a treat—let it rest for awhile, and listen to it sing.

Among other strategies, I do not deprive myself of dessert, so long as it does not contain gluten or casein. While it not a simple task to find such desserts, you can do it if you are creative. See pages 44 and 158 for starters. There are many delicious fruit combinations, and Vietnamese cuisine offers other dessert choices as well.

My pursuit of the *Tao of Youth* has brought me to pay closer attention to my inner physical being than in the past. One day recently, after I ate a good grilled salmon in a restaurant, I heard a sigh from my stomach as I sat: "This feels very good, May." I could have sworn my stomach was talking to me. Earlier I paid attention only when my stomach was unhappy.

As a result of all these eating strategies, I have a lot more energy as well as a glow to my face. In addition to weight loss, the total strategy allows my body an uncompromised immune system. No longer are the antibodies in my lymphatic system attacking antigens (proteins); now they are free to fight real disease threats. And with the extra enzymes provided by my new eating strategies, my body can concentrate on other, for instance metabolic, functions.

The eating strategies of Key 1 affect all the other keys to the *Tao of Youth*, Key 5 in particular. (See Key 5 for soups that are particularly good for your skin.) The digestive system is like your thumb, one of the most important parts of the hand, the first key to the *Tao of Youth*.

Recently I have been conducting workshops—often with my brother Dr. Sam, my sister Cathy, and Gary, our alpha music man—for women who may wish to pursue the *Tao of Youth*. I've noticed that while many women are enthusiastic about implementing the eating strategies of Key 1, they face some hurdles.

My advice is start slow, give yourself permission to fail now and then, and do not become discouraged. Stop eating gluten and casein as best as you can, listen to the recommended music (see Key 4), and drink the Oolong tea until you feel ready to take additional steps on the path. Then, try the juicing or some of the other recipes. To implement all the eating strategies, much more the whole *Tao of Youth,* is a mind switch from what you have been conditioned to for many years. Be gentle with yourself.

I have received many e-mail messages from women starting on the *Tao of Youth*. Many are creating new recipes and enjoying good results. Gary Hovda, our music partner, says he would never go back to his old ways of eating. Many women are interested in the workshop because they know that when you go back to nature—through following the ancients and adopting some of these more recent strategies, you restore your body. And your healthy eating will show in your face and your body and your spirit.

Gary's Story

Gary is 56 years old. Sam and I met him about two years ago. He started taking relaxin (see Key 2) at that time. Gary listened to the diet information we gave him but did not fully implement it until February of 2006. Since then he has lost more than 20 pounds, and his clothing is down a couple of sizes.

Gary has always been aware of diet, exercise, and fitness. He kept his weight at a normal range until he reached age 50—his body just naturally maintained a comfortable weight. Then to his dismay, he began gaining weight and a fullness in his upper body and face. Nothing he tried seemed to reduce it.

For many years Gary was a vegetarian. He bought and ate organic foods, and he read all the labels. He even implemented macrobiotics, though looking back he realizes he gained weight over the years when he mainly ate wheat, dairy, a few vegetables. Influenced by the food industry's promotion of "healthy" dairy and whole-grain products, he hadn't realized that these foods caused his fullness and extra weight.

Gary did not resist the idea of eliminating wheat and dairy from his diet. He understood the science behind Sam's theory, but he felt that because he was of Scandinavian descent and his cultural intake included high amounts of wheat and dairy products, his digestive system had evolved to tolerate them. He now knows he was "addicted" to both; they were his comfort foods.

Only when he gained more weight after age 50 and saw that it did not just "come off" with his normal routine did Gary begin to accept the "fact" that people fill out as they mature and simply must dress strategically dress to cover it. He became proficient at doing that but found it embarrassing to buy XL shirts and a pants size he never thought he would reach. Since almost everyone else his age was rounding out and most of his relatives had the same body shape, he convinced himself it was normal.

Because Gary provides an important element of the *Tao of Youth* lifestyle—the music—he accompanied Sam and me to Hong Kong in January 2006. Along the way we chatted about diet and exercise. He began to eat, enjoy, and understand Chinese food as well as to drink the tea we recommended. He continued this upon his return to the United States, though he sometimes responded to his wheat and dairy addictions. Still, he started to lose weight, about a pound per week.

Gary was running out of enough Chinese recipes to keep him happy with the variety in his eating. So I introduced him to "Five-Grain Rice," which helped him change his eating patterns. Finally he had something to replace the wheat that had satisfied him.

Gary then switched as well to rice-milk substitutes for dairy products, becoming wheat- and dairy-free. The weight still came off at about a pound a week, but the fullness in his gut, face, and upper body disappeared, and he returned to the size he wore before turning 50—from XL to M within a couple of months. He no longer dresses strategically.

Not only is Gary's weight back to normal, but also his energy has returned and his skin tone is 10 years younger. He maintains a wheat- and dairy-free diet totally from choice and not because he is on a diet. He has discovered many delicious and satisfying wheat- and dairy-free recipes. He prepares and cooks most of his own food but also has explored for and found wonderful meals at restaurants and delis. He eats and loves Chinese food but has found foods to enjoy from many other cultures —Mexican, Greek, Italian, other Asian countries, even from among the fresh Norwegian foods.

The *Tao of Youth* has become a life journey for Gary. He understands Sam's theory of water weight, but it is no longer just theory—he lives it and has reversed something that most people consider normal. He eats the recommended diet with supplements, maintains an exercise program that includes yoga and movement classes with some resistance and cardio training, and he listens to *Tao of Youth* music. He is amazed at how many people ask him how he maintains his earlier weight and such a youthful appearance. Most important, Gary enjoys his life again.

How to Flush Out Net Water Weight

We recommend the following natural methods, which may be used indefinitely, to flush your body of net water weight. Used together, they are particularly effective. Reduce or eliminate your consumption of gluten (in grains) and casein (in dairy products) before proceeding. During flushing, you may expect an increase in the volume, frequency, color, and odor of urination. The overall flushing process will take several months.

If you wish to flush a lot of water from your lymphatic system, drink 6 to 12 ounces of fresh-squeezed fruit juice together with 8 to 12 cups of Oolong tea, For maintenance, drink the fruit juice in the morning with a cup of tea and the rest of the tea throughout the day, brewing 1 or 2 teaspoons at a time. Following are the basic recipe for a healthful juice drink and instructions for brewing the tea.

Basic Juice Drink

Juicing is a delicious way to get the nutrients beneficial to your health and well-being. And raw fruits and vegetables provide natural enzymes that slowly degrade "foreign" proteins—the partially digested antigens that become trapped in the lymph nodes. I make this fresh juice every morning as part of my healthcare routine.

    4 small carrots or 2 big ones
    1 apple
    1 pear
    ⅓ cup frozen fruit

1. Juice the first three ingredients in a juicer to make 8 to 12 ounces of juice.
2. Pour the juice into a blender and add frozen fruit.
3. Blend, drink, and enjoy.

Add or change fruit to change the favor: plums, pineapple, cantaloupe, honeydew, cranberry, grape juice, or any fruit in season. Frozen fruit available in most grocery stores includes mixed berries (blueberries, raspberries, blackberries), mixed fruit, and strawberries. Other frozen fruits are fine, but these berries have the most riboflavin.

How to Brew Oolong Tea

Oolong tea is partially fermented (green tea is not fermented; black tea is completely fermented) and retains enzymes from the fermentation process helpful in flushing net water weight. Choose Oolong tea picked from the top of the mountain—there the tea produces more enzymes in the colder and more hostile environment.

> 1 4-cup teapot
> 1 to 2 tsp Oolong tea for each 2 cups of water

1. Heat the water and pour it over the tea to fill about one-third of the teapot.
2. Wait 10 or 20 seconds, and pour out the water completely to rid the tea of caffeine and dust.
3. Pour hot water again into the teapot until it is full.
4. Brew for 2 minutes. Pour the tea into any container and enjoy.

Brew Oolong tea two or three times from the same leaves, but for each brewing add more time—2 minutes at first, 4 minutes the second time, and 6 minutes the third.

Five-Grain Rice

Sometimes you just yearn for carbohydrates—to replace the bread and pasta or desserts you probably ate before. Five-grain rice and/or a steamed sweet potato easily satisfy that yearning as they provide natural-fiber antioxidants, balance blood-sugar levels (by not turning carbohydrates so quickly to sugar), and flush water from your system. Five-grain rice satisfies my need for carbs enough that I rarely crave the snacks that make my stomach feel puffy and my joints ache.

I'll admit it's taken me awhile to get to where I can say no to my brother-in-law, who loves his bakery goods and often offers them to me. But feeling and looking better is worth the switch. And you can make this dish as tasty as you want it to be. See the next page for rice and bean variations.

> 1 cup brown rice
> 1 cup Chinese red rice
> 1 cup white rice
> 1 cup beans of choice (soaked overnight)
> 4 cups water
> Pinch of salt
> Dash of oil

1. Soak the rice and beans overnight depending on the consistency of rice you prefer.
2. Bring water, salt, and oil to a boil.
3. Add all the rice and beans.
4. Simmer on low for 50 minutes (or less if you have soaked the rice).
5. Let stand 10 minutes before serving. Serve hot or cold.

Add a little flaxseed oil just before eating or stir-fry with fresh herbs. For variation, add a few dried shitake mushrooms and a small handful of dried Chinese goji (also called lichi or wolfberries), lotus seeds, and/or red dates.

For five-grain rice, use any combination of rice (brown, red, black, white, or wild) or other grains without gluten plus dried beans—black, black-eye, small red (not azuki), and mung. Those are my favorites. I like the beans for their flushing abilities and for their taste when combined with the grain, but there are many others. Don't be afraid to experiment. Just keep the ratio of 70 percent rice and grain to 30 percent beans and other ingredients. Though there are not five grains in the recipe, the name is traditional for recipes for any mixture of grains, not necessarily five.

Five-grain rice freezes well; it's easy to wrap and carry along a ball of rice for lunch. Many Chinese stores and co-ops offer five-grain rice, but the mixtures rarely include beans. It's more fun to try combinations and find out what you really like.

Good Healing Soups

For centuries, Chinese people have enjoyed nutritious soups with healing herbs. The people in southern China drank these soups when I was a child, and they still do. I now find them helpful to digestion and to flushing the lymphatic system. We usually do not eat the solid parts of soup but drink only the broth. It soothes the stomach and intestines, especially on days when we have not been eating well. The broth rests the stomach, nourishes and replenishes you. For a perfect healing soup:

1. Put the other ingredients in the pot after the water is boiling. This will prevent them from sticking to the bottom.
2. Use clay pots for making soups, as they are best for cooking over low heat for a long time. You can find clay pots at many Asian grocery stores.
3. Scald all meat with boiling water before putting it in the pot.
4. Avoid adding cold water once the soup is on the stove. Cold water makes hot meat contract and the proteins in the meat harder to digest.
5. Use high heat to bring and keep the soup at a boil for half an hour; then simmer over low heat for two to three hours depending on the particular recipe.
6. Add salt only after the soup is done. This prevents the proteins from solidifying and ensures good flavor.

Lean Pork Soup with Tomatoes and Potatoes

¾ lb lean pork (shin), rinsed and scalded with boiling water

1 to 2 medium tomatoes, washed and cut into pieces

3 medium potatoes, peeled, cut into pieces, and rinsed

2 oz goji (lichi or wolfberries)

12 red Chinese dates (seeded)

12 cups water

1. Bring water to a boil.
2. Put all the ingredients into the clay pot; cook over high heat for 20 minutes.
3. Reduce heat and cook for 2 hours.
4. Season with salt and serve.

Goji or Chinese wolfberries, an ingredient used in many soups and some herbal prescriptions, help flush water from the body. They taste almost like raisins. Chinese dates—different from the Middle Eastern dates most Americans are used to—have a soothing effect. Both are inexpensive and available in any Chinese grocery store.

Lean Pork Soup with Apples and Pears

13 oz lean pork

2 apples

2 pears

3 dried figs

1 oz sweet almonds

1 oz bitter almonds

12 cups water

1. Rinse all the ingredients.
2. Core and quarter the apples; core and halve the pears.
3. Cut the pork into four pieces and scald them with boiling water.
4. Bring the water to a boil.
5. Put all ingredients into the clay pot, and cook over high heat for 20 minutes.
6. Reduce to low heat and simmer for an hour.
7. Season with salt and serve.

The sweet or southern almond and bitter or northern almond (kernels of peach and apricot pits) nourish the intestines and stomach. Chinese groceries carry them.

Cooked Vegetables Salad

1 lb asparagus, cut into 2-inch pieces

1 lb (young) green beans, with tips broken off

3 yellow beets

1. Blanch asparagus for 2 minutes; plunge it into ice water.
2. Separately blanch green beans for 3 minutes; plunge them into ice water.
3. Marinate the vegetables separately with the following for 1 hour or at most 2 hours before serving. (You may cook them the night before.)

    2 to 3 T soy sauce

    1 tsp honey

    1 tsp roasted sesame-seed oil

4. Cut the yellow beets into slices. Stir-fry for about 8 minutes with:

    2 tsp cooking oil, such as canola oil

    2 cloves garlic, sliced

5. Add the following to the beets to taste. Put them into a container and refrigerate to serve with the other vegetables when you wish.

    1 tsp sugar

    2 tsp vinegar

6. Arrange asparagus on one end, yellow beets in the center, and green beans on the other end of a serving dish or platter. You and your guests will lick the platter clean!

Chocolate Coconut (Milk) Custard

Don't even think about giving up dessert when there are such healthy alternatives as the following gluten- and casein-free treat. Serves eight.

1 cup coconut milk
2 T butter (the only dairy product that's virtually casein-free)
3 T Ghirardelli Sweet Ground Chocolate and Cocoa
2 egg yolks
2 whole eggs
½ cup maple syrup
¼ tsp salt
2 tsp vanilla extract

1. Heat the coconut milk to just below a boil. Turn off the heat and take the pan off the burner. Stir in the chocolate powder and butter.
2. Beat the egg yolks and whole eggs together. Add the maple syrup, salt, and extract.
3. Pour a little of the hot milk mixture into the eggs to warm them. Stir and continue this process until you've added all the coconut mixture.
4. Divide the custard among eight ramekins, and place them in a baking pan containing a one-inch layer of hot water.
5. Bake the custards 20 to 25 minutes (or longer, depending on your oven) at 325 degrees F. They should be a little soft in the middle when you take them out. If you cook the middle until it is completely done, the custards will lose their tender texture. Cool, then refrigerate until serving time.
6. Dust the top of the custard with Dutch cocoa powder if you like.

Building Your Health Capital

People attending our *Tao of Youth* workshops frequently ask about how or what food supplements to take. Aggressive marketers approach us in many ways, pushing this or that. One explains why you should take a certain product; another recommends something else. Confusion reigns, and some people opt to take nothing at all.

Dr. Julian Whitaker's thoughts about why you need a multivitamin (page 48) provide a beginning framework for a food-supplement regimen. After reading many wellness books, I've discovered few other guidelines. And with Sam's help, I've devised the following approach.

In brief, three vital functions—the circulation of the blood, the reproduction of cells, and glandular production—together determine a person's "health capital." When these three play well, the orchestra that is your body makes beautiful music. When these functions fail or are not in synch, discord and chaos result.

Artery/Blood Health

An individual in good health circulates 250 billion red corpuscles, 15 billion white corpuscles, and 500 billion platelets daily, each renewed at its own pace. These corpuscles, in plasma, or serum, constitute the blood that feeds, protects, renews, and preserves your body.

Plasma, a thick liquid, functions as a coagulator. When you cut yourself—inside or outside—blood coagulates so that you don't lose too much. Plasma also contains other substances that defend the body. The corpuscles, suspended in plasma, move, change, destroy, and reconstruct themselves in an endless effort to maintain harmony, constantly renewing your life.

The blood vessels (arteries and veins) through which the plasma, red blood cells, white blood cells, and platelets flow are networks of tubes totaling 100,000 kilometers to and from the heart, which is the engine of the body, the pump. When the blood vessels are not healthy, arteriosclerosis, or hardening of the arteries, develops and makes them rigid. With atherosclerosis, the yellowish deposit of cholesterol on artery walls gradually wears them out. When a morsel of fat detaches, a clot may catch in the shrunken artery, stop blood flow, and deprive the cells of oxygen, which then die (coronary thrombosis).

All the systems of the body count on healthy blood, vessels, and blood flow, so anything you can do to monitor and maintain their good health is wise.

Cellular Health

The cell, capable of creating life and of reproducing itself, is the basic building unit of the body. It responds to two simple laws: anabolism—the construction of the elements necessary for life—and catabolism—the elimination of waste. A complete cell consists of membrane, and, floating inside it, cytoplasm, as well as organizers known as organelles. These active agents reflect the perpetual motion of life—the endocytosis vesicle provides absorption of food, the lysosomes provide digestion, and the mitochondria provide oxidation, all to nourish the cell and provide its energy. The chief organelle is the nucleus or root of life, containing genes, chromosomes, DNA—the entire program of your existence.

The slightest disturbance in the relationship or function of these components, in the balance of nutrients they receive, affects your health and equilibrium. Lack of magnesium, for instance, makes you tired. Vitamin A makes your skin soft; vitamin E prevents the formation of fat in your blood vessels. Keeping the balance is key.

What you eat supports the health or dysfunction of your cells. Eating unsaturated fatty acid (vegetable fat) vs. saturated fatty acid (animal fat), for instance, determines how information passes through and between the cells. Too much saturated fat makes cellular membrane inflexible, which impoverishes cellular exchange. Fish oil, olive oil, and camellia-seed oil nourish the cellular membranes, which control the equilibrium, "breathing," and waste elimination of the cells. Free radicals—unstable atoms—destroy the genes and destabilize the environment of a cell. When you're young, free radicals don't matter much (enzymes neutralize their negative effect), but age often provokes a drop in needed enzymes. Replacing them with supplements or food supply can make the difference. Antioxidants (notably selenium, zinc, vitamins E and C) defend against the damage of free radicals by eliminating their oxidation.

Glandular health

Less is generally understood about glandular health, but my brother, Dr. Sam Yue, has made a start with the study and use of a third major reproductive hormone—relaxin. (See Key 2). His research has included study of the endocrine system as important to healthy aging.

We define the glands in question as endocrine—"secreted within"—because they secrete hormones directly into the blood. Efficient and subtle messengers, the hormones oversee and stimulate the body's development through their cohesive influence on cells. Many glands—suprarenal, testicle, thyroid, pituitary, and so forth—secrete hormones.

The principle gland, however, is the pituitary, which secretes hormones that stimulate other glands—the thyroid, the suprarenal, a man's testicles, and a woman's ovaries. The pituitary gland secretes a hormone (vasopressin) that regulates water and another (prolactin) that causes lactation. The distribution of glands and the hormones they secrete occurs in a hierarchical manner.

Everything starts with your brain—the brain seats your consciousness. Or more precisely, it seats the nerve center possessed by all vertebrates—the hypothalamus—situated at the base of the brain. Here lies control of sleep, mood, instincts like fear, thirst, hunger, excitement, sexuality, and aggression—the elementary, active aspects of your life.

In the hypothalamus, a series of amino acids begins circulating in the blood, setting out to inform the pituitary gland. The amino acids transmit the messages sent to other glands through the intermediary of the blood and coordinate the release of hormones.

The pituitary produces hormone for direct use, such as growth hormone and one regulating glucose, as well as stimulating the thyroid, ovaries, testicles, pancreas, and suprarenal gland. The pineal gland, in the center of the brain, secretes melatonin, which helps you sleep.

As you age, gland function decreases and may not provide the secretions needed for well-body functions. And that's where food supplements come in.

Why Take Vitamins?

According to Julian Whitaker, M.D., editor of *Health and Healing*, few people eat a healthy diet, low in fat and refined carbohydrates and emphasizing whole rather than processed foods and at least five servings of fruits and vegetables daily. Only about 20 percent of us eat fruits or vegetables rich in beta-carotene.

Even if you try to eat in a healthy way, fertilizers, pesticides, storage, and cooking methods decrease nutrition in the foods you eat. And exposure to water and air pollution, mercury in dental fillings, preservatives, aluminum in cookware and antiperspirants, and other toxins takes a toll.

Our nutritional needs are greater than what the food supply delivers. Think of vitamin and mineral supplements as insurance against the inadequacy of a modern diet. A multivitamin is the foundation of any supplement program, one of the best things you can do to enhance energy, maintain a healthy heart and immune system, and live a more active life.

The sources, potency, and quality of nutrients vary, so read the labels. Look for the sources, or forms, of vitamins (indicated in parentheses after the name of each). Minerals are better absorbed in chelated form, meaning that they are bound to amino acids or other substances making them more available to your body. Watch for synthetic fillers that hinder absorption, induce allergies, or upset digestion. Some contain sugar, food coloring and flavoring, or additives such as chlorine. Make sure you get the specific nutrients you need in the amounts you need (see following).

Why We Suggest Food Supplements

Sam and I have noticed that many people are confused about food supplements. There are so many products and there's so much advice—it's intimidating! Those who come to our workshop may already have started on a vitamin regimen, but they want to understand more about the topic.

We have come up with a strategy of three simple steps. Everything we recommend falls in the three categories of building and preserving your health capital—blood and vessel health, cellular health, and glandular health.

Taking Your Vitamins

- Take multivitamins in divided doses. Your body usually secretes what it doesn't use within hours. Replenish nutrients through the day for maximum benefits.
- Don't worry about precise division.
- Take supplements at the same time every day, so that it is easy to remember.
- Always take supplements with a meal or snack to avoid an upset stomach and to assist absorption.
- Sometime a large dose can cause uncomfortable reactions, If you have a lot of gas or get diarrhea, for example, when you are taking Vitamin C, reduce the dosage for a week, build it slowly, and take divided doses.
- For best results, take supplements immediately following exercise (with food).
- Organize the supplements you'll need for the week. Put each day's dosage in a sandwich bag or pill container. You'll save time, and you can take them with you.
- Remember that supplements do not make up for an unhealthy lifestyle. Eat and drink well, exercise, relax, and sleep.

The first step is to start on a good multivitamin and mineral regimen. Sam likes Dr. Julian Whitaker's Forward Plus Daily Regimen®. I like Dr. Garry Gordon's Beyond Chelation® Dietary Supplement Program. I also like Life Extension's Super Booster. If you stack up the labels, you will find these programs similar. They all put together for you what you might have to guess about otherwise. Basically, they contain vitamins A, B and C complex, D and E, a mineral complex, plus omega-3 and omega-6 essential fatty acids and others. These multivitamin programs are more expensive than those found over the counter, but they are designed for maximum purity and absorption. (See opposite and following for multivitamin dosage.)

The second step is to supplement enzymes for digestive purposes, related to Key 1 in particular. The majority of our workshop participants have some type of digestive problem. As you age and when you are in menopause, you lose 40 percent of your enzyme production. On top of that, Americans, especially, tend to eat hard-to-digest foods in large quantities. That makes your digestive system work overtime, compromising enzymes needed for other purposes. Tibetan medicine teaches that hundreds of diseases start with poor digestion. Make sure your digestive system is vital.

Beyond avoiding foods containing gluten or casein, be sure to eat foods full of enzymes. Supplementing enzymes comes in when you find that even that is not enough. Sam sees many patients with this problem and so has put together a program for them and our workshop participants to supplement enzymes. Being on this regimen has made a world of difference to me. (See pages 138–39 for enzyme sources and dosage.)

The third step is to supplement hormones and provide food supplements and herbs specific to your family history. For example, you might take CQ10 if your family has history of heart disease, or acetyl-L-carnitine and alpha lipoic acid if there is a history of Alzheimer's. Take Biolaxin™ (porcine relaxin) to prevent or delay the onset of adult-onset diabetes or diabetes type 2 if both your parents suffer from this disease. The males in our family have all died of strokes, so Sam takes nattokinase for stroke prevention.

Everyone is different. With the results of baseline blood, hormone, and bone density tests and knowledge of family medical history, you can decide with your physician whether and what hormones and supplements you need. See page 62 for information on a blood-test panel and pages 53–54 for supplements beyond multivitamins and minerals. See Key 2 for the missing link in hormone replacement.)

Recommendations for Daily Vitamin and Mineral Intake

Instead of basing your nutrient intake on the Recommended Daily Intake (RDIs) of the Food and Nutrition Board of the Institute of Medicine, look for a multivitamin providing optimal health benefits and helping to prevent age-related disease.

Neutralize free radicals and their damage to cells (atherosclerosis, cancer, Alzheimer's disease, cataracts, osteoarthritis, and immune deficiency) with antioxidant vitamins A, C and E, carotenoids (especially beta-carotene and lycopene), and the mineral selenium.

- 2,500+ mg vitamin C (build gradually over a week, spread daily intake)
- 800 IU vitamin E (as tocopherols or tocopheryls; D-alpha-tocopherol rather than DL-alpha-tocopherol; the L after the D indicates a synthetic)
- 5,000 IU vitamin A (retinol)
- 15,000 IU beta-carotene

B-complex vitamins are essential for proper functioning of your nervous system, including mental functioning, and for metabolizing homocysteine, which damages arteries and reduces the integrity of vessel walls.

- 50 mg BI (thiamine)
- 50 mg B2 (riboflavin)
- 100 mg B3 (niacin and niacinamide) (may cause flushing of the skin if taken on an empty stomach; look for a supplement combining the two forms)
- 50 mg B5 (pantothenic acid)
- 75 mg B6 (pyridoxine)
- 100 mcg B12 (cyanocobalamin)
- 400 mcg folic acid (especially important for women of child-bearing age, to prevent spina bifida or other neural-tube defects in offspring)

(continued on the next page)

Vitamin D aids the absorption of calcium and phosphorus, helping to prevent decreased bone density and a predisposition toward fractures in the elderly. The ability to manufacture vitamin D from sunlight decreases with age.

- 400 IU Vitamin D
- Essential fatty acids reduce the incidence of high cholesterol, stroke and heart attack, angina, high blood pressure, rheumatoid arthritis, and cancer. (If you have heart disease, lipid disorders, or diabetes, discuss taking Vitamin D with your physician before doing so).
- 1,000 mg fish oil (with 180 mg EPA and 120 mg DHA, omega-3 fatty acids, and 125 mg omega-6 fatty acids from borage oil)

Optimal human nutrition requires 22 minerals involved in the composition of bones and blood, functioning of cells, and composition of body enzymes. The most important major minerals are magnesium, potassium, and calcium.

- 500 mg magnesium (cofactor of more than 300 enzyme reactions, important for protein formation and DNA production, helps turn food into energy, prevents muscle cramps, maintains intracellular potassium levels, blocks entry of excessive calcium, increases metabolic efficiency of the heart, decreases insulin resistance in diabetics, and helps prevent heart attacks, high blood pressure, heart arrhythmia, asthma, and kidney stones)
- 99 mg potassium (helps maintain water balance and distribution, muscle and nerve cell function, heart function, and kidney and adrenal function)
- 1,000 mg calcium (most absorbable forms are citrate, malate and ascorbate; builds bones and teeth, helps vital functions, assists normal clotting)

Trace minerals assist metabolism:

- 200 mcg selenium (organic, helps prevent heart disease and cancer)
- 30 mg zinc (necessary for proper action of hormones, immune function, wound healing, vision, male sexual function, and skin health)
- 200 mcg chromium (chromium picolinate for best absorption; essential for carbohydrate control and insulin action, beneficial in treatment of diabetes, weight loss, and reduction of blood lipid levels)
- 2 mg copper
- 10 mg manganese

Food Supplements

A good multivitamin is the base:

- Capsules or softgels are usually better than tablets.
- Usually store-bought vitamins are hard to digest and absorb.
- Dark yellow urine indicates good absorption.

Biolaxin™ (relaxin) 20–40 mcg (1–2 tablets) twice daily

- Prevents insulin resistance (delays onset of DM type 2 up to 10–15 years)
- Increases microcirculation to the organs and skin
- Promotes release of endocrine hormones
- Promotes sleep
- Promotes energy and stamina

Acetyl-L-carnitine (500 mg) twice daily with
Alpha lipoic acid (300 mg twice daily)

- Improves brain function
- Possibly prevents Alzheimer's disease

Coenzyme Q10 (30 mg two or three times daily)

- Improves heart and musculoskeletal function (a must for those taking statins to lower cholesterol/prevent muscle weakness; the water-and-fat-soluble form (Q-gel) is three times more absorbable than regular CQ10)
- Works with acetyl-L-Carnitine and alpha lipoic acid to reduce fatigue

D-ribose (2 tsp twice daily) and/or ATP (125 mg twice daily)

- Improves total energy (at cellular level) for those with chronic fatigue

Chelated calcium (180 mg) and chelated magnesium (100 mg two or three times daily)

- Prevents osteoporosis and supports the integrity of muscle contraction and relaxation (shown to reduce colon polyps and possibly cancer)
- Check body pH (7-8 or higher) to assure absorption of calcium. Chelated forms are easier to absorb.

(continued on the next page)

Glucosamine (500 mg twice daily)
Chondroitin (500 mg twice daily)
MSM (methylsulfonylmethane) (1 gm twice daily)
Celadrin® (Cetyl myristate) (350 MG twice daily)
- Take in combination or individually to promote joint health.

Fish oil or Omega 3 oil (EPA/DHA)
- 1 gram three times daily to promote general well-being and prevent inflammation
- 2–3 grams three times daily to prevent joint and other inflammation

If you cannot tolerate fish oil, use one of the following in similar dosage:
- Flaxseed oil, primrose oil, borage oil

Saw Palmetto (160 mg twice daily or 320 mg once daily)
- Prevents benign prostatic hyperplasia (BPH) in men
- Lycopene, beta-sitosterol, pumpkinseed extract, pygeum, and DIM complex (diindoylmethane 100 mg)

L-arginine (500 mg two to three times daily)
- Used with relaxin, controls IBS (irritable bowel syndrome)

Lutein (20 mg daily) and bilberry (6 mg daily), usually in combined form, and/ or Zeaxanthin (258 mcg daily)
- Prevents premature lost of eyesight

Nattokinase (65 mg or 1,000 FU—fibrinolytic units— twice daily)
- Dissolves fibrin to prevent strokes (If you are taking Coumadin®—or its generic warfarin—consult with your physician first.)

Super Greens (1 level tablespoon or number of capsules suggested on the label) (made of freeze-dried sprouts of wheat, barley, oat, rye and other vegetables)
- Assists digestion of gluten and other proteins naturally
- Supplements the required 5 serving of daily vegetables
- Provides natural fibers and nutrients

Key 2

Understanding your internal

fountain of youth

A Cinderella Story

Our path to the discovery of Key 2 is a Cinderella story. Sam and I are like fairy godmothers. As we asked many questions about ways to balance the hormones of women undergoing menopause, we found a hormone—relaxin—that most people have never heard of. And we responded to her weeping.

I call relaxin the Cinderella hormone—she has stayed in the kitchen the past 60 years. Though she is the hardest working of all the female reproductive hormones, she is kind and gentle, and almost no one has recognized her importance. Relaxin assists many body functions and helps your other hormones work well together, but she rarely gets any credit.

Relaxin's stepsisters—estrogen and progesterone—are related to her but do not have the same mother. They have different characteristics and behave in a different manner from relaxin; they have a dark side. The outside world has embraced the two stepsisters, and some people have exploited them by making them seem more potent than they are.

55

The prince (you) is unhappy and confused by the two stepsisters being sold as the answer to your happiness. Never quite satisfied with the two stepsisters, the prince still looks for the right mate—and decides to host a ball to find just the right one.

Sam and I—the fairy godmothers?—want Cinderella (porcine relaxin) to be known so that the prince can be happy. We know that in this case there is still another sister, a beautiful one who looks almost like Cinderella (human relaxin, a maternal twin, is nevertheless for this use an imposter). The real Cinderella must appear at the ball so that the prince can find the one he truly loves.

Cinderella comes to the ball, dances with the prince, and he falls in love with her. But at midnight Cinderella must leave, and she drops a glass slipper. The prince picks it up and uses it to find for the real Cinderella. Who will fit into her delicate shoe?

As the story goes, the stepsisters (estrogen and progesterone) try on the shoe, which fits neither of them. The almost twin (human relaxin), who looks like Cinderella, also tries it on. She looks so much like Cinderella that the prince thinks she may be the one. Alas, she has a bunion and cannot fit into the shoe.

Finally the true Cinderella (porcine relaxin) tries on the slipper. It fits perfectly. The prince hums with happiness: The kingdom (your body) is in balance; there is perfect harmony once Cinderella comes into the fold. They live happily ever after.

Searching for a Magic Wand

My sister Cathy is a year younger than I. As children, we shared the same bedroom for many years. We have our differences, but we are close. About 12 years ago she asked me whether I was interested in learning more about menopause even though we had not yet reached that part of our lives. "We could prepare for it," she said. There were not so many books on the topic then as there are now.

I agreed she had a good idea, and together we developed a strategy. She selected newsletters on the topic, and we divided the tasks of reading them, sharing information, and asking our brother, Dr. Sam Yue, to clarify confusing medical terms and some of the more technical issues. We subscribed to newsletters put out by physicians interested in alternative medicine. We set out to find out about estrogen, progesterone, and everything we could about menopause. We faxed to each other any ideas that made sense.

The first book we read was Anne Louise Gittleman's *Super Nutrition for Menopause*, on taking vitamins and food supplements as a means of alleviating the symptoms of menopause. We implemented her program and found it helpful but continued our research.

I had asked my gynecologist how I should prepare for menopause. She said, "You are not there yet. I just checked your blood test, and your FSH is not high enough for me to recommend your taking Premarin®. When it's high enough, I'll let you know."

As she showed me out, I thought "Whoa, that's way too little information for me to decide such an important issue!" Now I know that FSH stands for follicle-stimulating hormone, which increases when estrogen is low. But that wouldn't have made much difference—what I questioned was the wisdom of Western HRT (hormone replacement therapy).

I decided to take on another search: To learn about the Chinese herbs that help eliminate the unpleasant adjectives of menopause that Suzanne Somers has called the Seven Dwarfs—itchy, bitchy, sweaty, sleepy, bloated, forgetful, and all dried up! I read literature on all types of Chinese and other conventional herbal remedies for those symptoms—herbs such as don gui, black cohash, and others.

My sister subscribed to a newsletter by Jonathan Wright, M.D., and I read Dr. Susan Lark. Both provided information helpful in making right choices for ourselves. I have since met Dr. Wright and his wife, Holly, at antiaging conferences and other alternative-medicine meetings. We got to know the two even better when they flew to St. Paul to have my brother Sam treat her painful shoulder.

I found Dr. Wright most informative. The first to introduce natural, bio-identical HRT, he has more than 20 years of experience in his field. I highly recommend his book *Natural Hormone Replacement* to women over age 45. And his special report, *New Secrets Every Woman Needs to Know,* is a must read. (See Sources & Resources.)

After reading *New Secrets,* Cathy and I decided we would not replace our hormones with Premarin®. Dr. Wright explains it well—Premarin® is a combination of estrogens concentrated from horse urine—principally equilin. But there are some important differences between horse and human estrogens. For example, the effect of equilin on the lining of the uterus is up to a thousand times stronger than that of human estrogen. (This provides a clue as to why Premarin® may increase the risk of uterine cancer.).

I cannot emphasize enough that the balance of hormones is a crucial piece of the well-being of every woman—as well as of how well she ages. And the balance is important for many reasons beyond relieving menopausal symptoms. In Key 1, we discussed facilitating well-balanced digestive and lymphatic systems. Well, all of the hormones are interrelated, and balancing your endocrine system is important too.

A whole new medical practice—antiaging—has evolved over the past 12 years. Before that, there was no certification of doctors for such a specialty. This new specialty has taken HRT to a new level—to the balancing of hormones in the body, way beyond replacement during menopause. There are large bodies of continuing antiaging research. The layperson must be informed to make the right choices.

When anyone mentions hormones, most of us think only of estrogen and progesterone. But there are many families of hormones, and they all work differently within your body.

The American media have, in many instances, misguided women and their physicians with news about HRT, probably because reporters and their editors do not understand all the implications of what they broadcast. In July 2002, for instance, the Women's Health Initiative (WHI) abruptly halted its HRT research and instructed all women on HRT to discontinue taking the hormones. I was not surprised because my sister and I had done our research and decided long before not to take Premarin® or Prempro® (a combination of estrogen and progestin). These were the most widely prescribed hormones, the ones used in the WHI study.

We set about learning what we could about HRT, and you will make the best decisions for yourself if you do too. There is no mystery to understanding it if you put your mind to it. My sister and I are laypersons. Yes, we have a brother who can answer many of our questions and ask even more. But don't forget—he is a man. And it was only at our urging that he came to help us solve some of our problems. He learned from us as well, and now his practice includes some HRT for menopausal women.

Life Extension's *Disease Prevention and Treatment,* especially the chapter on female HRT, explains in simple terms the mainstream- and alterative-medicine points of view. I chose natural hormone therapy for the early or perimenopausal years. Because of our southern Chinese diet, my sister and I do not have severe menopausal discomfort. The natural HRT concepts we use came about as a result of studies in Asia showing that many of the menopausal disorders of the Western countries are nonexistent or minimal in women of the East. The Eastern diet relevant to this discussion includes a large amount of soy products and a low intake of fat.

Hormones are messengers, carrying a signal from one organ to another or from one organ to a group of cells. For example, estrogen promotes growth of the endometrium (lining of the uterus). Any hormone sends its message by "locking on" to the cell wall of a target organ at a place called the receptor site. Once locked in position, it changes the cellular metabolism of that particular cell by turning on or off certain genes that code for the manufacture of specific proteins. The genes of the cells translate these messages to produce the code effect—in this case, the growth of the uterine lining to prepare for the implantation of a fertilized egg. (Estrogen plays other roles in other parts of the body.)

I found this information helpful in coming to a decision about Western HRT. For a part of the body to function well, the structure of the cell walls must be such that they accept the hormone molecule completely. The cell-wall structure depends on the kind of food one eats, particularly the kind of fat.

Imbalances of dietary fat change the three-dimensional structure of the cell wall (the receptor site). The hormone comes along to transmit a message but does not fit into the cell wall correctly. The message is minimized or a larger amount of the hormone is required to achieve the same result. Think of the receptor site as the lock and the hormone as the key. If the lock changes, the key will not fit into the lock; the door will not open, or it will open only after many trials. Taking in a good balance of saturated and unsaturated fats (including omega-3 oils) and eliminating trans fats goes a long way towards ensuring receptive sites of good quality.

Any hormone that has transmitted a message must then be deactivated. This is what happens when we detoxify something. The body changes the hormone; then it deactivates the hormone and excretes it.

In the case of estrogen, deactivation takes place in the liver through a process called glucoronidation or conjugation. If the process is not working well, active estrogen may circulate through the body unnecessarily (and may aggravate, for instance, the metabolism of a cancer). Any chronic digestive or liver condition, any imbalance of healthy bowel bacteria, leads to this situation.

Taking care of the digestive system may seem a long way from hormone balance. But as I learned from the bold characters announcing on the walls of a Tibetan medicine manufacturing company in Yunan in June 2006: "Hundreds of diseases begin with failure of the digestive system." The digestive system is important indeed. We spent a lot of space explaining Key 1 so that you could know alternatives for keeping it in balance.

Another thing you need to know is that there are many hormones in your body and they all talk to each other. Various kinds of hormones gather into separate families according to their functions. Understanding their differences is important to learning how to keep them in balance—the best way to age well.

Finding a doctor who will help you monitor hormone balance is important. For example, estrogen and progesterone work together in the steroidal family as part of your reproductive system and other body functions. Insulin is part of the polypeptide insulin family (as are relaxin, IGF-1, and so forth), which affect, with all the other hormones, all your other body functions as well. The thyroid hormone has its own family. There are others, too.

All these hormones and families of hormones have different characteristics. You do not need to know all of their characteristics for an understanding of Key 2, but be aware that there are many hormones in many families, all with different purposes. Using relaxin, for instance, does not metabolize, or float around your body after its work is done, in the way that estrogen does. Adverse news about one hormone does not mean you should not take any at all. Learn what you can before you throw out the baby with the bath water.

We present Key 2 to help you understand your reproductive systems just as we tried to help you understand your digestive and lymphatic systems and water versus fat weight. We take away the mystery; we set out to understand it and give you a report. We use the same methodology to get to the hidden facts; we share our findings so you can make better decisions for yourself.

After reading Dr. Wright's special report, I found out that Chinese physicians were the first to use bio-identical HRT—for the emperor and his court. They evaporated urine from women in their late teens and early twenties, then combined the crystalline residue with herbs and sweet gums for the use of the women of the imperial court. They did the same for the men of the court, with urine from young men. Those who took these preparations noted an antiaging, rejuvenating effect on their skin, a major boost in energy, and an improvement in sex drive.

I don't suggest that you do what they did but present them as an example of people in ancient times trying to find antiaging remedies. Today we have many ways to improve the aging process without eating dried urine. We have not yet reached the understanding we desire, but when we do, Cathy and I will decide on the best course of action regarding Eastern HRT. Together we are still pursuing the antiaging part of the search.

About five years ago my brother suggested that Cathy and I participate in a study. He wanted to determine the levels of hormones in our blood at our current ages and use those figures as a baseline for recording later levels. He also wanted to follow bone density. We discovered that our Western, conventional physicians do only limited blood work because the insurance companies cover only standard tests. They do not cover extensive measurement of hormone levels. We decided to pay for the other tests ourselves, and because of that investment we have been able to get a sense of where we are and how to replace what we are missing. The list of tests in the blood-test panel we recommend includes IGF-1, estradiol, FSH, LH, TSH, T3, T4, DHEA, testosterone, and prolactin levels, plus bone density, colonoscopy, and mammogram. You can find the list in the Life Extension Foundation's magazine each month. (See Resources). The blood-test panel will provide a wealth of information useful in making decisions about your health.

Another book by Suzanne Somers—*The Sexy Years*—is also full of useful information. I especially like the chapter in which she interviews Diana Schwarzbein, M.D. What I understand from her research is that it is best not to replace a hormone if it is not low or missing, but to mimic normal physiology as much as possible and to track hormone levels and their effects. These makes sense to me, and my sister and I have been following these guidelines.

Finally, Cinderella

After a few years of searching for the best answer to our perimenopausal and post-menopausal problems, I found myself seeking a new career. I was running a software company when it suddenly took a new direction and I was out. It would have been natural for me to look for another company to run or to find other familiar work such as with a financial firm.

My brother Sam had been trying to get my attention for a couple of years. I had brushed him off because I was on a fast track with little time to see or understand what he was doing. He asked me to help him organize and run a new company, mentioning that he had discovered a major pregnancy hormone—relaxin—with great implications for wellness. I was not sure at first about accepting his offer, but I decided to pursue the same kind of due diligence I would for any career choice. The first step was to interview him.

I share with you my process of understanding to let you know why I decided to partner with him on this project. The first topic that I wanted to ask him about was this thing called relaxin. I did a little research before going into the interview, and this is what I found:

The use of relaxin can be traced back thousands of years to the Chinese culture, where the consumption of certain pig organs, high in relaxin, was used to reinvigorate human organs and promote good health. Relaxin was first discovered and investigated in the United States in 1926, when Frederick L. Hisaw, a soon-to-be Harvard researcher, reported the muscular relaxation benefits of porcine relaxin injections in female guinea pigs. Relaxin, identified as a polypeptide hormone belonging to the insulin family, has been found in the females of all species studied.

During the 1950s and 1960s the Federal Drug Administration (FDA) approved porcine relaxin, sold under the brand names Lutresin, Cervilaxin, and Releasin. They were used extensively for treatment related to cervical ripening, premature labor, in vitro fertilization, pulmonary fibrosis, peripheral arterial disease, glaucoma, and scleroderma.

In 1962, the Kefauver-Harris Drug Amendments mandated that every FDA-approved pharmaceutical product, in addition to proving safety, prove efficacy. Since porcine relaxin had been used safely and effectively for 18 years and because of the expense of clinical studies to prove efficacy, the company that produced Lutresin chose to circumvent the mandate by taking the FDA to court. The company ultimately lost this legal battle and, as a result, porcine relaxin was taken off the market in 1972 due to "unsubstantiated efficacy"—but not to safety issues.

To date more than 1,500 research articles have been published on the impact of porcine relaxin on human physiology. Despite this body of evidence, porcine relaxin has been virtually ignored in the United States due to a lack of communication between the scientific and medical communities and to changes in pharmaceutical economics as a result of the 1962 Kefauver-Harris Drug Amendments.

During the 1990s, Dr. Sam Yue observed that many of his female patients with multiple health issues (fibromyalgia) reported that their symptoms began or worsened after menopause or hysterectomy. These patients also reported that their symptoms went into remission during pregnancy but returned one or two months after delivery. Intrigued, Dr. Yue began to look for a substance produced naturally in the body that could account for his observations. His initial research focused on the two most well-known female hormones: estrogen and progesterone. But he could establish no link between either or both hormones and his patients' reports.

Dr. Yue continued his research, which ultimately pointed to the hormone relaxin. During pregnancy, relaxin production increases almost tenfold. After menopause or hysterectomy, relaxin levels dramatically decrease. While he initially focused on the benefits of relaxin in treating fibromyalgia patients, his continuing research indicates relaxin is beneficial in the treatment of a wide range of health and wellness issues.

What Sam Found

How did you discover this hormone?

Multiple fibromyalgia patients reported that their many symptoms related to FMS (pain, muscle spasms, IBS, insomnia, lack of energy or fatigue, concentration, and others) seemed to subside or disappear during pregnancy. After delivery, most of the symptoms returned within a month.

This set me in search of the mysteries of pregnancy and, after reading many research articles on relaxin, I came to the conclusion that, indeed, relaxin was the reason these patients felt good during pregnancy. After additional research, I came to believe that relaxin has many useful functions outside pregnancy and that many FMS patients exhibit the symptoms of menopausal women, though in a more severe form. Many of the symptoms of menopause seem related to a deficit of relaxin or to an insufficient balance of relaxin, estrogen, and progesterone. Thus relaxin probably would be helpful to menopausal women.

Why don't most people, including those in the medical community, know about relaxin?

Somehow, after 1972, relaxin fell off the radar screen of most clinicians, and despite the urging of basic researchers, few physicians pay any attention to this little-known though well-studied hormone. Connetics Corporation, a pharmaceutical firm, for one, spent tens of millions of dollars trying to revive human relaxin as a commercial drug. But in a quirk of nature, supplemental human relaxin (the imposter twin) just doesn't fit into the receptor sites in the body the way porcine relaxin (the true Cinderella) does. Attempts failed, and relaxin again fell into obscurity. At this time, nine of ten physicians do not know that there are three hormones related to the menstrual cycle and pregnancy, or that the third major female reproductive hormone is relaxin.

So, in a nutshell, what is the commercial history of porcine and human relaxin?

Porcine relaxin was available from 1950 until 1972. Attempts to commercialize human relaxin in the 1980s and 1990s failed. Now BAS Medical, a small start-up is again trying to commercialize human relaxin.

Which organs produce relaxin? How is relaxin different from the hormones estrogen and progesterone?

The major relaxin-secreting organs are the ovaries, then the uterus, placenta, and possibly some others. Relaxin belongs to the insulin family of hormones and does not affect the estrogen and progesterone, or steroidal, family. Unlike steroidal hormones, the insulin hormones do not metabolize as the body quickly deactivates and sloughs them off.

Have there been scientific studies of this hormone?

In addition to thousands of basic scientific studies delineating the effects of relaxin on individual organs either in vivo or vitro in animals, there were many human studies of porcine relaxin from 1950 to 1972. Since 1972, there have been multiple double-blinded placebo-controlled studies of human relaxin related to the induction of labor, scleroderma, and other conditions. (See Sources & Resources for a list of these articles.)

What are some of the physiological functions of relaxin outside of pregnancy?

One major benefit of relaxin is its enhancement of microcirculation in the vascular system. Relaxin may in this way promote the efficient functioning of many organs through an increase in blood supply. One of the first signs of aging is a decrease in the function of some organs from a progressive lack of microcirculation; relaxin restores it. Relaxin benefits many other functions, but its enhancement of microcirculation, which enhances many other functions, is the main benefit.

What effects of relaxin have you observed in your patients?

Research has shown that relaxin increases coronary flow by stimulating nitric oxide production. This promotes the dilation of blood vessels and, as a result, improves microcirculation. Relaxin also influences the secretion of insulin-like growth factor-1 and growth-hormone secretion of the pituitary gland, increasing cell growth and differentiation. Relaxin stimulates collagen synthesis and secretion and increases the deposits of new collagen, especially in the presence of estrogen. Collagen, found in all types of connective tissue in the body, provides strength and support for the tissues.

The epidermal cells and hair follicles of the skin contain receptor sites for relaxin. Based on clinical study and experience, we have found that through the induction of growth factors, collagen-remodeling effects, and increased circulation, relaxin helps to normalize cell and collagen turnover. This results in more elastic and flexible collagen and thickening of the epidermis.

In addition, relaxin facilitates the integrity and quality of collagen in the connective tissues. As a result, the skin is rejuvenated; it becomes translucent and radiant, taut and more youthful in appearance, in a reflection of how well the internal environment is functioning.

What are some of the side effects of relaxin?

I hesitate to call these side effects—they're more like side benefits. Relaxin seems to reduce the need for other medications. Relaxin changes the insulin resistance of cell walls and thus reduces the requirement for insulin. For patients who take insulin, relaxin may reduce the insulin requirement by 30 to 40 percent, with a result of hypoglycemia if insulin intake is not reduced.

Relaxin releases serotonin from the central nervous system, so for patients who take SSRI-type antidepressants, the dosage should be adjusted downwards. And it provides other benefits such as the reduction of pain, spasm, insomnia, and other symptoms for which medication also should be adjusted.

––––––

Lackin' Relaxin? Sam's Notes on Related Disease

Through the years, I have been surprised that relaxin, particularly porcine relaxin, has made such a profound difference in the lives of some of my patients. Unfortunately, most of the basic studies so far have focused on the use of relaxin in pregnancy (it is often called the third pregnancy hormone). But like estrogen and progesterone, relaxin has other physiological functions; these have not been studied enough, especially in relation to disease.

No studies of disease related to deficits of relaxin seem to exist. But I believe the lack of relaxin produces several diseases, including fibromyalgia (or FMS, which I mainly address here) and adult-onset diabetes. The regular ingestion of relaxin appears to effect total body changes in patients with fibromyalgia.

Relaxin ingested over a course of three to six months by patients with fibromyalgia appears to reverse organ failure or the beginning of failure associated with FMS. Patients with adult-onset diabetes taking relaxin, particularly porcine relaxin, experience relief of the symptoms of diabetes in addition to an easing of insulin resistance. Relaxin also improves the health of the parts of the body involved in the diabetic process.

Human relaxin produces physiological changes only when administered at pregnancy levels, but porcine relaxin administered at $\frac{1}{10}$ to $\frac{1}{15}$ of that dosage produces change enough to relieve the systemic problems of many patients with diabetes and FMS. The potency of porcine relaxin is clearly superior, so I use that at this time.

I have treated patients with fibromyalgia for as many as 20 years and so have been able to observe their appearance and overall well-being over long periods. In my observation, FMS patients age 40 to 50 percent faster than the healthy population. They often lose hair and teeth, they gain weight easily, their organs fail, their skin becomes patchy, and they experience difficulties with their organs. Patients in their thirties often complain of the bowel-related problems more commonly experienced by people in their eighties and nineties.

As many have noted, people with diabetes also age faster—30 percent faster than the norm. Given that relaxin reverses many symptoms of FMS and diabetes and returns those patients' age progression to normal, I can only hypothesize that taking relaxin generally blocks the aging process. Since the first sign of the aging process in the general population is related to microcirculation—just as it is in patients with diabetes and FMS—the process of aging may occur at least in part because of a lack of relaxin. If so, the ingestion of relaxin may help delay inherited type 2 diabetes as much as 10 to 15 years, thus preventing premature aging.

Taking relaxin also reverses negative changes in microcirculation and much of the aging process. The antiaging community has advocated the use of growth and other hormone replacement to protect patients from premature aging. This is especially popular in Europe and Southeast Asia, where almost every hormone—testosterone, estrogen, progesterone, growth hormone, even cortisol (hydrocortisone) and thyroid hormone—is balanced to its optimal level. But physicians, including antiaging physicians, have grossly neglected relaxin.

Once you replace relaxin, which produces a harmonious effect, rebalancing other hormones (usually with lesser amounts) is necessary. For example, many studies show, and my observations in clinical practice confirm, that relaxin releases growth hormone. In addition, it releases serotonin and melatonin and modulates other hormones from the pituitary.

When relaxin's role is ignored, balancing hormones requires a larger and more persistent effort. But if relaxin releases and modulates many of these hormones to a point that adjustment becomes unnecessary or minimal, patients need much less supplementation to have a healthy, vibrant life as they age. What I have seen in my pain clinic leads me to believe that relaxin is an antiaging hormone. Folks in their nineties move with the bodies of 60- and 70-year-olds; people in their sixties and seventies have the bodies of most in their forties and fifties. This may directly relate to the effect of relaxin on the function of internal organs (for example, by improving circulation and thus the more efficient production of hormones).

Relaxin is not a panacea, but it does have multiple physiological functions. Relaxin, for example, may make much smaller doses of estrogen effective for the optimal functioning of women on estrogen replacement. But relaxin is countered by testosterone in men, who might require a larger dose. This has to do with receptor sites, a subject beyond this discussion but with tantalizing prospects for antiaging in men as well as women.

In conclusion, relaxin is an antiaging hormone appropriately used by healthy persons to maintain wellness, to prevent early or premature deterioration of organs, and even, perhaps, to prevent the development of FMS and diabetes through the reduction of insulin resistance. These are good things, at least for individuals reaching advanced age. Relaxin makes a person feel better because of the release of serotonin and melatonin. And it reduces the need for antidepressants and sleeping medications. Further, relaxin has a synergistic effect with many hormones—those affecting the menstrual cycle and the ability to conceive. This is probably related to how relaxin regulates estrogen and progesterone. It also appears to regulate ovulation and to facilitate sperm swimming up the cervical canal.

For all its virtues, physicians do not recognize relaxin as a major female hormone for reasons unclear. In fact, 90 percent of physicians do not understand or recognize that three hormones affect women's menstrual cycles or know that the third hormone is relaxin. Relaxin nevertheless has huge potential for increased wellness in our aging population. Together with other hormones it can provide a vibrant life without postmenopausal problems for women—and a life without the difficulty of age-related decreases in hormones for men.

Further, relaxin has a significant beneficial effect on patients suffering from diabetes, as well as on those with Alzheimer's disease, who become calmer and more reasonable, easing the workload of their caretakers. Recently the link between Alzheimer's disease and diabetes has begun to become clear. One study has found that the brain tissue of an Alzheimer's patient does not utilize glucose as well as that of a healthy individual. In fact, researchers have labeled Alzheimer's disease "diabetes type 3," indicating that Alzheimer's is a diabetic disease manifested in the brain. The study shows that everyone generates plaque formation in the brain as rapidly as Alzheimer's patients, but Alzheimer's patients do not seem to clear plaque as quickly or easily as healthy individuals. Whether plaque is a direct cause or secondary manifestation of another disease process is unclear. Some researchers believe Alzheimer's is related to an inability to utilize glucose well, thus hindering the clearing of plaque.

These ideas are an exciting development given my observations of individuals with FMS, who are prone to diabetes and Alzheimer's disease and who, I believe, suffer from a lack of relaxin. Though appropriate studies are still to come, the possibility of one day preventing or delaying onset through the early ingestion of relaxin by individuals prone to Alzheimer's disease offers great hope indeed.

———

After talking with my brother Sam about this hormone, I realized how much this discovery was like the discovery of what to do about water weight. The answer was right before our eyes—he rediscovered this hormone. And its implications are far-reaching.

Relaxin, estrogen, and progesterone are the three hormones produced during the menstrual cycle, yet women have been advised to replace only two of them. In fact, for those prescribed estrogen (Premarin®) alone, only one is replaced. After reading many different articles about HRT, we found only a few (European) physicians who have recommended replacing relaxin. We found only one article published in the United States—"This Relaxin Is Relaxing Too Long" in *Science* 295 (January 2002).

Relaxin is one of the most important considerations in keeping us healthy because it is a master hormone that balances the production of other hormones and provides many other benefits through improved microcirculation. It is not a major hormone like insulin, adrenaline, or cortisol (stress hormone), crucial to such life-sustaining functions as a regular heartbeat, blood pressure, and maintaining pH balance (blood acidity/alkalinity). If you are missing any of those, you will quickly become ill and die.

Instead, relaxin is a minor hormone like estrogen, progesterone, testosterone, and DHEA. It deserves their status yet has been ignored as a source of general wellness and prevention for premature aging. My sister Cathy and I have decided to incorporate relaxin into our HRT regimen, and SKY BioHealth Solutions now manufactures and makes available porcine relaxin as a food supplement. (See Sources & Resources). For women during and after menopause, Dr. Yue recommends one tablet daily, progressing to one tablet twice daily, for maximum benefit.

A Few More for the Road

Cathy and I have been tracking our T3, T4, and TSH (indicators of thyroid) levels for several years. Our earlier levels were considered normal, so we did nothing with this hormone until we read Dr. Jonathan Wright's newsletter about how the "normal" Western diet does not include nearly the amount of iodine that Japanese women ingest. Generally they consume at least 12.5 mg of iodine daily, while Westerners consume only 1 mg. Dr. Wright recommended a product called Iodoral®, which is a combination of iodine and iodide (as potassium salt) for the best absorption.

I decided to implement his recommended course because about 30 years ago a benign tumor necessitated the removal of one of my thyroid glands. My physician at the time said that one thyroid gland was sufficient to produce enough hormone the rest of my life. My T3, T4, and TSH test results were "normal." But if I have only one thyroid gland that has been producing hormone for many years, I thought, surely it could use some help as I age. I began taking Iodoral® and since then have felt a lot better—wonderful, in fact.

I did not have time to renew my supply of Iodoral® before a recent trip to China and so went for three weeks without it. Soon I noticed I felt generally anxious and that I lacked my usual energy. When I returned I renewed my supply, including

Iodoral® in my supplement regimen. The difference is incredible. Iodoral® helps my single thyroid gland produce enough thyroid hormone to keep me at my best.

I have learned through these last 12 years of preparing to age well that we consumers need a different mindset—we must ask about and learn about how aging affects us and about what we can do about it, instead of passively accepting the information (or lack of it) provided by the health care industry and drug companies. And now that I have mastered, for myself at least, the symptoms of menopause, I wish to take my health to another level . . . into the field of antiaging.

One thing I have learned is that when test results are declared normal, you need to know what normal means. The norm for age 60, if that is your age, is not necessarily the one you wish to match. Take the case of bone mass. We lose bone mass starting at age 35 so if you are normal for that age group, you are already in decline. I want to do better than that. I want my bone mass to improve so that it is 15 to 20 percent above the norm for my age group—the optimum.

This is a new way to look at wellness. It may be controversial to expect such a result. But if we can be younger through eating well, keeping our digestive and lymphatic systems in good shape, and balancing our hormones, why shouldn't we reach that goal—and even look beyond?

Dilman's Theory of Aging

A few years ago my brother Sam and I attended an antiaging conference. There Ward Dean, M.D., introduced us to the Dilman's aging theory. (Dr. Dean published a series of special reports on this theory in *Vitamin Research News* in 1999.)

Vladimir Dilman, a Russian gerontologist published his aging theory in 1954—in Russian, so his theory is little known outside Eastern Europe. He theorized that aging is caused by a progressive loss of sensitivity by the hypothalamus and related brain structures to negative feedback inhibition.

What does that mean? As you age, the endocrine system does not respond as well to what once were adequate levels of hormones in your body. It works like the thermostat that controls the temperature in your home. A finely tuned thermostat maintains your quarters at a narrowly defined, comfortable temperature. When the thermostat (the main control of hormone secretions) wears down and loses sensitivity to the temperature (level of hormones in the body), the house temperature (level of secretion) becomes more varied and uncomfortable since the thermostat does not kick on and off as it should.

The endocrine system becomes dysfunctional as the body ages, and this dysfunction brings on metabolic changes. The changes include:

1. a reduction of glucose tolerance
2. an increased level of insulin in the blood or serum
3. an elevated level of lipids in the blood
4. the onset of diseases such as obesity, diabetics, cancer, hypertension, depression, fatigue, and atherosclerosis.

Dilman believed that the use of antioxidants alone does not extend maximum life span (the free-radical theory of aging) because it does not address the neuroendocrine (glandular) causes of aging. Sam and I agree that focusing on cellular health (relying on the free-radical theory of aging by taking antioxidants) without also looking after your glandular health will not promote healthy, graceful aging.

Key 1 addresses cellular health through ingestion of the right foods and maintenance of a healthy digestive system. Key 2 addresses glandular health. Through treating and observing his patients, Sam has come to believe that relaxin plays the role of modulator (maestro) of the endocrine system. Relaxin somehow gets a message to the hypothalamus, restoring an adequate hormone-release sequence to the pituitary gland and others (thyroid, adrenals, testes or ovaries, and thymus). Again, your body is like an orchestra—every instrument is important to playing beautiful music, important to the melody as a whole.

Our workshop helps women to understand their baseline blood-test panels and bone-density tests for a better understanding of their health. We recommend they become members of the Life Extension Foundation so as to receive its informative book *Disease Prevention and Treatment* as well a year's subscription to its monthly magazine. The foundation also offers blood tests for monitoring progress.

So you supplement your diet and monitor your hormone levels with blood tests. Those tests do not include levels of relaxin. In fact, Sam has found no commercial test capable of determining levels of relaxin because any level of relaxin is relatively low. As a result, he has asked Immuno-Diagnostic Company in Germany to help develop a test for both human and porcine relaxin levels, which will be available soon.

Since everyone is different, we advise you to work with your physician to arrive at a yearly monitoring program that fits your needs. With baseline blood results you can look for appropriate food supplements beyond the basic multivitamin/mineral program. My brother has provided a list of food supplements and herbs suitable to those with various needs. As mentioned earlier, I chose Iodoral® for my thyroid plus L-arginine and relaxin for my GI tract. The males in our family have all died of strokes, so Sam follows a regimen addressing that potential problem. Those with diabetic parents might address glucose tolerance, and so forth. (See page 51–54 in Key 1 for more food-supplement strategies.)

Just Out: Keeping Your Eggs in Your Basket

I read in the October 2006 issue of *O, The Oprah Magazine*, an article by health writer Barbara Seaman titled "Keeping All Your Eggs in Your Basket." Seaman pointed out that, for women, conventional thinking is not always wise.

For example, consider the impact of a less invasive lumpectomy versus a debilitating radical mastectomy—the almost automatic treatment of breast cancer into the 1970s. Journalist Rose Kushner persuaded President Jimmy Carter through the National Institutes of Health to fund clinical trials investigating whether lumpectomies worked just as well as the radical procedures. They did. Seaman stated that the Halsted radical mastectomy was "the greatest standardized surgical error of the century."

And what about taking the ovaries? Federal data from the late 1990s show that 78 percent of women aged 45 to 64 undergoing hysterectomy also had healthy ova-

Relieved

I have been May and Cathy Yue's Pilates teacher for many years. At age 43 I suffered night sweats, mood swings, and exhaustion. Upon Cathy's suggestion I joined Life Extension (LE) and requested a female blood-panel test. It showed I was physically way beyond my age, postmenopausal in many areas. LE suggested urinalysis and— because my younger sister was diagnosed with breast cancer—an estrogen check.

Noel Radcliffe, M.D., a local holistically certified physician, looked at my test results, ran more tests, and encouraged me to have the urinalysis. LEF then referred me to Dr. Jonathan Wright's lab for the 24-hour test. This involved two weeks of taking my body temperature and providing data about what I ate, including supplements. After the results were in, a physician at Wright's Tacoma Clinic asked me in for a consult but agreed to do it by phone. He went over all of the test results and recommended specific supplements to bring up my numbers.

Shopping for supplements at Whole Foods Market®, I received a great deal of help from a clerk who suggested a vitamin called Doctor's Choice for 45-Plus Women by Enzymatic Therapy, containing everything I needed. That clerk is one of few people I have found to know much about women's hormones. My local physician added the test results to my medical record and followed up with blood work after I had been on the vitamins for several months. She prescribed a progesterone cream that, together with the supplements, resolved my symptoms.

The doctors I had seen previously had been trained to look for disease and didn't know what to do with me if I didn't have one. Once I had antibiotic-induced clostridium difficile, and they did not know that I could simply balance the bacteria in my colon to get rid of it. They wanted me to take on a high-powered antibiotic and stop nursing my six-week-old baby (because of the antibiotic). Cathy and May brought me an intestinal flora supplement that cured me in 24 hours. And the relaxin they gave me relieved my post partum depression, allowing me to teach as usual.—Meggie

• • • • •

The medical system is far from perfect. Ultimately each one of us is in charge of our own health. Meggie's new physician, open to alternative medicine, continues to learn. Meggie realizes she can't know it all but that she must know the whys of health and not just the symptoms of disease, that she is responsible for much of what ails her, and that she can do plenty to make it better.

ries removed. The conventional thinking? Without ovaries they would not be at risk for ovarian cancer. William H. Parker, M.D., a clinical professor of the David Geffen School of Medicine at UCLA, published a study in the August 2005 *Journal of Obstetrics and Gynecology* that made the gynecological community take a second look at what it had been doing.

Dr. Parker, who once believed in taking perfectly good ovaries for reasons of prevention, took a second look when writing *A Gynecologist's Second Opinion*. His editor, Janine O'Leary Cobb, questioned his position on oophorectomy. She had heard too many women who lost their ovaries complain about their loss of energy, concentration, and interest in sex and living.

Janine Cobb's questions prompted Parker's initiation of a clinical study with Michael Broder, M.D., and a team of other physicians and scientists. They took data from dozens of published studies, using a mathematical model to estimate the impact of ovaries in versus ovaries out.

Based on the model, 10,000 women aged 50 to 54 undergoing hysterectomy would have 47 fewer cases of ovarian cancer by age 80 than a similar group of women keeping their ovaries. The oophorectomy group, however, would suffer 838 more deaths from coronary heart disease as well as 158 more deaths due to hip fracture. Forty-seven women would be spared ovarian cancer—but only at the cost of more than 900 lives—of women whose hearts and bones failed without the normal hormonal support that their ovaries supplied.

The bottom line? Unless a woman is at high risk for developing ovarian cancer based on genetic testing or family history, there is no advantage in the removal of her ovaries.

This case in itself suggests we should not be intimidated. The doctors speaking to conventional methods may be mistaken or at least may not be thinking in terms of your particular case. We, women especially, may have to question protocol to obtain better solutions.

I did a head count of immediate friends, finding that six of them have had hysterectomies. Only one had cancer. The rest chose the surgery to relieve a tough menopause. A physician suggested the surgery to my sister after a year of extensive bleeding. I went through a rocky period, too. But there are many ways to make life easier without removing your reproductive organs.

The use of birth control pills has created a whole new set of conditions that women of previous generations did not endure. Sam has observed in his thousands of patients that the onset of many symptoms of early aging is related to the overuse of birth control pills or hysterectomy. One friend told me after her surgery that she felt her essence as a woman had disappeared. Her nurse practitioner said she hears that every day from women who have had hysterectomies. As far as I'm concerned, the fountain of youth is in my ovaries. Why get rid of them unless I have no other choice?

To take this particular line of thinking a step further, Sam and I remind you of the three major pregnancy hormones produced by the ovaries—estrogen, progesterone, and the Cinderella hormone, relaxin. We speculate (because of studies on animals, see Sources & Resources, pages 173–75) that the missing hormone related to heart muscle and the collagen matrix of bone is not estrogen or progesterone but relaxin. In any case, we must keep looking beyond the conventional wisdom, asking and pushing for the facts and studies, so that we can choose the right course for ourselves.

And Just One More

Today is December 15, 2006. A headline on the front page of the *Minneapolis Star Tribune* (over an AP story by Marilynn Marchione) touts a decline in breast cancer since the year 2003. The 7.2 percent decline came a year after a federal study linked the risk of breast cancer with heart disease and other problems. Within months, many women stopped taking estrogen and progesterone. Experts now believe the decline in breast cancer is related to the much lower use of hormone replacement therapy (HRT).

Why did all we women fail to question the validity of using Premarin® earlier? Why did we need this many years and this many lives to pass before changing our strategy? I am so glad my sister Cathy and I prepared ourselves before menopause, that we chose not to use the HRT our gynecologist suggested, that we sought alternatives in handling the symptoms of menopause.

We are coming into a new era of defining wellness and health practice. It is up to each of us to explore and seek new information, to take back the power, ask questions, and perhaps make new assumptions. We can't depend on conventional wisdom without question. Our very health depends on finding answers of our own.

Key 3

Understanding posture: What are you doing at the gym?

Muscles that Flex

Everyone knows exercise is good for you—or is it? Who would guess that many of the exercises we do at the gym promote premature aging? After you reach a certain age, such exercise will do nothing but wear out your joints—and your muscles. Your posture and walking gait are more important to your long-term health, to the activities you wish to pursue—and they give away your age. An understanding of posture, and how it changes with age, will help you figure out how to correct it while you still have time. So this key is really about posture, not exercise.

For several years, my brother Sam has told me that about 80 percent of the pain experienced by his patients occurs in two areas of the body. He's worked to figure out why that is so and to find a remedy for their pain. Many of the aches and pains of these younger men and women are also the complaints of "normal" older men and women. The reasons and remedies for their pain perhaps apply to the aging population in general.

Close your eyes and visualize walking behind an 80-year-old man and an 80-year-old woman. What is their stride, how do they walk and stand, in comparison with 20-year-olds? The elders probably have hunched backs, perhaps walk with a shuffle. The 20-year-olds walk with straight backs and a longer, stronger stride. Why the difference? And why do 80 percent of Sam's patients experience pain in the neck-and-shoulder or hip-and-back areas—the areas we see askew in the aging population before us?

We know that as we age, muscles get tighter. Does that have something to do with it? Can we do something about the tightness, the lack of flexibility? Can we reverse the tightness that's already there and bend with the wind again? Let's take a look at how we can keep musculoskeletal functions as close to those of a younger person as possible.

What Doesn't Work

I followed a certain exercise routine for some years, starting in my thirties.

I had inherited a hunched-over posture in my shoulder and neck area so had round shoulders and a tendency to dip my head forward when I walked. When I was a girl, my mother hollered at me to straighten my back every time we went out, and she had an irritating habit of poking my back as I walked beside her.

Let me tell you something about being the daughter of a mother from *The Joy Luck Club* era. After I read Amy Tan's book about her mother, I began to understand my own. Both of their lives were unstable during World War II, during eight years of fighting the Japanese, and during two migrations to escape Communist China.

Somehow this has meant that as their daughters, we must be perfect, must live with paranoia and impossible expectations. We are programmed to look and be at our best because they went through so much and they want to make sure we are prepared for every possible misfortune. I became quite aware of my little imperfection (poor posture) because my mother never stopped reminding me of it. I straightened my shoulders and back in her presence but went back to hunching my shoulders when she was not there—and I could forget about it.

I still remember my good friend Cecilia saying that my then-husband David asked her to remind me to walk with a straight back as the matron of honor at a friend's wedding. I tried many times to change my posture with little success.

Now I am older, doing Bikram yoga, watching myself in the mirror of the studio where I exercise. Bikram yoga specifically instructs the use of a mirror so that practitioners can easily watch their posts (positions) and bodies. I am proud to say I have since overcome my posture problem.

And I realize now that to maintain or move towards good posture, opening my shoulders for the moment my mother hollered was not enough. By the time I got back to my normal walking time, I was simply hunched over again. That hunched posture is almost a universal sign of aging—see that posture in those aging before you. All those years I had prematurely aged posture—no wonder my mother was disturbed by my stance!

About 11 years ago my brother discovered Pilates routines (at that time Pilates was not so popular as it is now: mostly it was used by dancers for injury prevention). My brother, my sister, and I attended a class conducted by a Pilates master. He explained the importance of a person's "core" and said that if you are working on your hips, for instance, you must work constantly to fill the curve in your back so that you can touch the floor. In other words, you tilt your hip and work on that motion to strengthen your core—and your posture changes. The hips govern upper/shoulder posture too.

Eureka! After years of poor posture, years of thinking I could never correct it and feeling inadequate about how I presented myself posture-wise (I closed my eyes to see dancers and wished I could stand as tall and straight), I was delighted to learn I could correct my stance with work on my hips and core. I immediately signed up for the class with my sister and my niece.

We have been doing Pilates once a week since then. Once I wanted to quit the big class for more individualized sessions, but my sister protested: "You cannot quit—Alicia [our niece] comes because we have all committed to doing this every week—for 11 years!" So I did not quit the group sessions, and my niece didn't either, and it has been gratifying to watch her grow up with Pilates. She was 11 when she began to exercise with us; she stopped only when she went away to college.

While I was doing Pilates with Cathy and Alicia, I also did other exercises at the gym—three or four times a week. There I took aerobic and cross-training classes. I was quite active and soon suffered many aches and pains. I found a massage therapist and took acupuncture treatments to rid myself of muscle pain.

About four years ago my brother introduced me to Bikram yoga after a trip to California. I tried a session and liked it very much though it was tough; I attended about once a week. Then I decided to do it three times a week—with no idea that I was overstretching.

All those years of running, aerobics, and cross training had turned my muscles tight and hard, especially on my left side. My right leg is about a quarter of an inch shorter than the other, and I favored use of my left side. The extra stretches of Bikram yoga (three times a week) had overworked my left leg and my piriformis muscle. (My brother told me later that it just snapped like a breaking rubber band.)

I had spasms of pain through my leg; I could not get out of bed; I could not move without sharp pain for five days. I was in bed for a week, and my brother the pain doctor was out of town for four of those days. When he came back, I begged him to do something, anything, to relieve my pain.

I went to his clinic for a Botox® shot in the piriformis; with the piriformis numb, the other muscles could relax and start rehabilitation therapy. I was going to quit the Bikram yoga because the whole experience had been so painful. Still, Sam said I should go back to the stretching and take it slow. My biggest problem is that I am driven to achieve (still trying to be perfect for my mother, I suppose) and take too little time for myself. That painful experience was a good lesson—now I have greater empathy for people who suffer.

I also gained insight into my muscular health in learning about what happened to my tight muscles—especially to the deep muscles around my hip area—when I did too much conventional exercise. For the past four years I have done no traditional exercise but have concentrated on motions that give me more balance and strength.

I am in the process of correcting the deep tight muscles that gave me so much trouble. It's taken me four years to be able to do most of the 26 poses of the Hatha yoga in Bikram yoga. Now small increments of change are important to me. I slowly stretch my muscles—for greater flexibility, strength, and balance.

What gives me joy now is to be able to go up and down the steps into and from the subway with no pain—just like a younger person. (I love to visit Hong Kong and New York and to be able to use their subway systems with ease.) Another great joy is to be able to lift my luggage from the airport conveyor belt with no problem—my core is strong and my body balanced. And I've noticed that I have so much more energy when I travel—my brother Sam has asked me to cut some activities because others cannot keep up with me. I have to laugh—all but Sam are younger than I.

If you follow such a regimen, you too can live an active life.

Posture, Aging, and Exercise: An Inquiry

Sam, what have you learned about posture from treating patients who have chronic pain?

In treating the muscle-related problems of these patients for 20-plus years, I have found that most of their pain is centered in two areas—the pelvic and shoulder girdles. Most pain in the lower back occurs around the pelvic area and radiates to the legs, sometimes to the middle back and abdomen. For those with shoulder problems, pain occurs mostly in the shoulder girdle, radiating to the neck and head, and from the head, to the neck, to the shoulders and arms.

Almost 70 to 80 percent of most patients' pain problems occur there, and if we treat that muscle-related pain, we eliminate most of their misery. Once the pain problems are eliminated, however, exercise and rehabilitation become an issue.

How do you treat the pain? And how does this apply to healthy individuals?

Many years ago I learned to inject botulinum toxin into the lower back muscles in what I call a psoas compartment injection. The toxin specifically numbs or relaxes the psoas and quadratus lumborum muscles on either side of the lumbar plexus (a network of nerves along the spine). After making many such injections, I was able to conclude that they relieve back-related pain for a prolonged period of time. Other kinds of injections, specifically spinal (epidural and facet) injections, do not relieve back pain as well as the psoas compartment injections, which suggests that the psoas and quadratus lumborum greatly affect the state of the lower back. That the injections relax those two muscles, significantly relieving pain, confirms that they play a part in generating pain in the pelvic girdle of the lower back.

With this in mind, I began to examine the cervical neck region to discover whether there was a similar structure within the shoulder girdle. I found that the scalene (anterior and medius) muscles play a role in generating pain in the shoulder girdle similar to those of the psoas and quadratus lumborum in the pelvic girdle of the lower back. Between the two scalene muscles is the brachial plexus reaching into the arms. This network of nerves plus the arterial and venous blood vessel comprise the brachial plexus complex, a neurovascular bundle reaching the arms through two muscles, similar in structure to the psoas and quadratus lumborum and the lumbar plexus between.

I began to inject patients in the neck through the brachial plexus. These injections affected cervical neck pain to a much greater extent than other spinal injections aimed at relieving pain in the same area. I was able to greatly reduce the pain by reducing patients' neck-muscle spasms with similar injections, including botulinum toxin.

Did those injections take care of the problem permanently?

No. I found that rehabilitating patient posture—so as to prevent potential future pain—remained a problem. With injections in the lower back or neck, my patients experienced relief for three to six months before the pain slowly returned. Then the cycle of pain-muscle spasm repeated itself.

I wondered what I could do to disrupt the cycles of pain and began to look into the relationship of the lower back girdle and the upper neck or shoulder girdle. How might posture (a result of repetitive and habitual use and adaptation of the lower back and shoulder girdles) predispose a person to injury—or prevent the full rehabilitation of muscles after an injury? I began to gather information on patient posture, mostly through observation and examination, in hope of learning how to eliminate posture defects so that my patients could rehabilitate themselves to the fullest extent.

What did you find?

I learned that the relationship between the pelvic and the shoulder girdles imparts posture and about how aging posture affects stride and gait.

Gait and posture reveal how old a person is. Or, to put it in another way, people judge a person's age (on first impression) by gait pattern and posture. And the exercise regimen currently practiced by much of the general public and medical profession results in poor posture and gait. Common exercises tighten, shorten, and eventually weaken the neck and lower back muscles, inducing posture and gait patterns that further tighten, shorten, and weaken the neck and back muscles. This vicious cycle contributes greatly to the premature aging of posture.

What other factors may predispose us to premature aging of the musculoskeletal structure?

First, gait and posture are influenced greatly by minor defects inherited from your parents. For example, one of your legs may be slightly shorter than the other, and your pelvic bone, particularly the major pelvic bone (the innominate), may as a result be smaller on one side than on the other. This gives you a tilted pelvis, which causes a slightly drooping gait in which you put greater weight on the shorter side when you walk. You can spot this postural defect and related gait easily if you take a moment to notice the people walking about in a shopping mall.

Other minor congenital defects include scoliosis (or curvature of the spine), usually found in the lumbar region but sometimes in the thoracic area. Scoliosis may be functional, meaning secondary to having one shorter leg, or real, if the legs are even and the scoliosis is real. Both cause a twisted spine that slightly skews the pelvis and posture to one side, inflicting wear and tear on those parts of the body before others. One-sided wear and tear causes premature aging of the posture.

Upon examination of the cervical neck area or shoulder girdle, patients exhibit many shoulder and neck variations (sloped shoulders, a thickened neck, a long and narrow swan-type neck, or shorter upper arm). In the case of a shorter upper arm, patients may shift the fulcrum (leverage) of the arms from shoulder to neck, resulting in a thick, full neck, or full clavicular fossa (in which the clavicles are not visible). Many swimmers and weightlifters attempting to strengthen their necks end up compressing the scalene muscle within the thoracic outlet, cutting off circulation in the upper right arm. This condition (it's sometimes called the "seventh cervical rib" syndrome) may also occur congenitally, with a longer seventh cervical rib serving as the compression point.

Such problems change both posture and gait. When you have a shorter leg or smaller hemipelvic bones on one side of your body, you tend to walk with a drooping gait. That gait wears the short or drooping knee more than the other, and the shorter pelvis wears the muscles on one side more than the other. These conditions negatively affect posture. The pelvis rotates in a slightly offset manner to adjust for the short leg, transferring muscle tension to the cervical and shoulder girdles, causing the opposite shoulder to rise.

Through the examination of seemingly minor defects that nevertheless cause damage, I have noticed that the pelvic and shoulder girdles are interrelated. If the pelvic girdle is not symmetrical, the shoulder girdle also becomes asymmetrical, causing the patient to walk with a funny gait. Rather than swinging the arms evenly, she swings them in an offset manner. With the muscles unevenly engaged, she develops asymmetrically in the areas of the lower back and upper neck. That may not matter much until she injures the lower back or upper neck area and begins to walk in a way that exacerbates injured muscles. Asymmetrical development, wherever it occurs, makes rehabilitation difficult.

The muscle from the pelvic girdle transfers asymmetrical tension up the cervical neck through the spinal muscles to the cervical region. Likewise, an asymmetrical shoulder girdle eventually results in an asymmetrical pelvic girdle. All these asymmetrical, or pathological, postures result in or affect pain within the pelvic and shoulder girdles. The knowledge gained from my experience in correcting posture, relieving pain, and rehabilitating patients with chronic pain applies as well to the health of the woman or man on the street.

How are the two pelvic and shoulder girdles related to each other?

The spine has several curvatures—a large, gentle S-curves from the upper thoracic to the pelvic area; the neck or cervical spine also has its own gentle S. The lower part of the cervical neck curves towards the front (the last part of the gentle S), and the thoracic spine curves toward the back, with the lumbar spine curved toward the front again. This S-curve of the spine (without the cervical neck region) in healthy individuals is relatively tall. The S-curve, in which the two girdles lie (shoulder girdle at the top of the S, curving back, and pelvic girdle at the bottom of the S, curving forward), is not compressed in healthy individuals.

So how does this apply to me?

Slow compression of the spine, as influenced by the pelvic and shoulder girdles, is a normal part of aging. Constant use of the muscles along the two girdles and any defects inherited from your parents over time affect the two girdles, the curvature of your spine, and eventually your posture.

As you age, you use the muscles in your lower back and neck in different ways, slowly rotating your pelvis forward and slowly shrinking your overall height through the compression of the S-curve of your spine. The pelvis tilts forward, the belly pops out in front, and the shoulders stoop forward. This process of normal aging, causes many older men to belt their pants above a waist shortened by compression of the S-curve or below a large potbelly.

As the spine shortens (or as the S-curvature compresses), you progressively become shorter, and your rib cage slowly descends until the last rib cage overlaps your pelvic bones.

Is the deterioration of aging different from that of your patients or from that resulting from minor physical defects?

Muscle deteriorates in the same way no matter what disease is behind the deterioration. If a person suddenly has a spinal cord injury resulting in paraplegia or a paralyzed leg, the muscles in the leg deteriorate rapidly, but the changes within the muscles are identical to that in a person suffering from multiple sclerosis or advanced age. The deterioration of the muscle of a person paralyzed from the waist down occurs within several months while that in a person of age 80 or 90 has taken decades, but the result is the same.

Aging results in muscle changes identical to those in patients with spinal cord injuries, multiple sclerosis, or any spinal or head injuries resulting in the deterioration of muscle. The masses of muscles are replaced partially with fatty tissue. They are no longer as dense upon examination by x-ray, they become more spastic (tighter), and the linings (fascia) enclosing the muscle fiber show ridges from contraction instead of the healthier, smooth surface. As muscles deteriorate, through disease or aging, they become tighter and pull down whatever they are attached to.

So as we age, gravity pulls the muscles and skeleton down with assistance from the muscles themselves, and posture changes. We lose height, we lose muscle mass, and we lose the flexibility of the musculoskeletal system, particularly in the joints—the hip, lower back, knees, and neck.

But it is a common misconception that this is an inevitable progression, that the muscles must deteriorate and gravity eventually pull your skeleton down, that you must lose height, flexibility, and range of motion. We all know of people of 80 years and beyond—perhaps a dancer or someone who practices Pilates—who stand straighter than many women in their thirties. Exercise that elongates the shoulder and pelvic girdle muscles can counter the effects of aging.

What kind of exercise? I already do a lot.

The "physical fitness" routines currently in vogue exacerbate and prematurely impart an elderly spinal configuration to those who undertake them. Most people, even specialists in exercise physiology, do not pay much attention to this problem; many recommend exercise that reinforces the tightening of muscles in the pelvic region, which pulls the spine forward, tightens muscles in the shoulder region, and causes the shoulders to stoop forward and compress the spine.

So what kind of exercise does work? Is it the same as for your patients?

Yes, but my advice varies from that of the majority of pain specialists and exercise physiologists, who ignore musculoskeletal fitness in emphasizing exercise for cardiovascular fitness. Most of what they recommend makes use of only a few of the muscles of the lower back, shoulders, and arms to get the heart pumping. Without musculoskeletal fitness, exercisers often prematurely fatigue and thus contract these muscles, compress the nerves, resulting in asymmetric pelvic or shoulder girdles and premature wear and tear. Whatever activity you engage in daily affects your posture and musculoskeletal health, so exercising to counter tight and spastic muscles in the pelvic and shoulder girdles is a good idea.

Gravity exacerbates tight muscles, slowly pulling the pelvic girdle forward and the spine down until a person assumes "elderly" posture. So exercise must address the flexibility of muscles in the pelvic girdle as well as range of motion for the spine and related pelvic joints. A flexible pelvic girdle, with full range of motion at the waist and lumbar spine plus flexible pelvic muscles, enables a less compressed S-curve. The corrected, more flexible pelvic girdle transfers its flexibility through the lumbar spine to the thoracic spine, allowing work on the shoulder and neck muscles to correct the compression as well as any extension of the neck and head.

The correction of unhealthy posture is long, slow, difficult work, as it is the result from many years—30 to 40 years for most people—of slow muscle adaptation. For example, some ophthalmologists who routinely do microscopic surgery develop severely compressed S-curves (particularly on the thoracic spine) from how they sit in front of the microscope when practicing their profession. To change this requires a significant amount of work on the pelvic region before work on the lumbar, then on the thoracic spine, can even begin.

What do you mean by musculoskeletal fitness of the pelvic and shoulder regions?

This means that a person has a full range of motion from the waist. For example, a fit person can bend over and touch full palms to the floor, which indicates full flexibility of the spine in the back. The fit person can bend backward without much of a problem and can turn sideways, rotating left and right. To achieve the full range of motion, all the pelvic muscles must be flexible.

The body is like a race car. You must tune it up before entering the race. If the car is not tuned properly, the engine breaks down. If your musculoskeletal system is not fit, you are prone to injury. Once injuries occur, they significantly affect and often injure other parts of the body. One sees this all the time in athletes—at least in the weekend athletes, who have pain in one knee, shift the body to adjust for the injury, and injure other parts so that rehabilitation becomes complicated and difficult. If you achieve musculoskeletal fitness, you will be able to engage in physical activity with much less incidence of injury, much less likelihood of lingering pain.

What kind of exercise will correct unhealthy posture and rigidity?

Some of the most "ladylike" exercises are the best for patients with chronic pain as well as for more healthy individuals. One that I recommend to patients is yoga; Bikram yoga is good for active people with few injuries, people engaged in physical activity for musculoskeletal fitness. Bikram and other types of yoga help to stretch and lengthen the muscles and increase motion in the joints for greater flexibility, strength, and power.

Other beneficial activities include the exercises of Joseph Pilates, a yogi himself, whose invented muscle movements and exercises initially were adopted by dancers, then by others around the world. Pilates work emphasizes the core muscles of the abdomen, which allow extended activity without fatigue.

Since we use the abdominal muscles and the flexor muscles of the hip in almost every activity of daily life, it makes sense to focus on increased flexibility in these regions. This means contracting or tightening muscles as they are lengthened, to give the long, lean muscle of a dancer rather than the tighter muscle of a football player.

Pilates exercise develops the flexibility of many of the hip and pelvic muscles and thus, eventually, of the cervical neck muscles. A complementary program of Gyrotronic exercise, consisting of rib-cage-muscle motions and flexion, extension, and rotational movement of the entire spine will also help. In addition, exercises like Tai Chi impart stability or balance through the gentle contraction of muscles and through motions shifting the exerciser's center of gravity.

What's the bottom line for the kind of exercise I do?

In general, Pilates, yoga, and Gyrotonic exercises are better suited for younger and more active individuals focusing on the core muscles and flexibility of the spine. Tai Chi may be more suitable for older and other perhaps less active individuals focusing on balance.

The important thing for any kind of exercise is that it tunes the body and provides flexibility, stretching the muscles to allow a full range of motion for the joints. To excel in sports activities without injury, the individual first must have musculoskeletal fitness. Those who primarily seek cardiovascular fitness are likely to injure themselves from asymmetric muscle use and to develop premature aging of the posture from repetitive, pejorative use of the neck muscles. They are likely to suffer joint difficulties and develop the asymmetric pelvic and shoulder girdles that result from premature aging.

One side benefit of good posture and muscle and joint flexibility is that even as you age, you will retain a good walking gait and appear to have an ageless body. If you walk like a young person, you will look young. You will also be able to engage in strenuous activity without pain or injury. You will act young as well. As for cardiovascular exercise, once your body is tuned up and you are able to maintain musculoskeletal fitness, any activity that keeps your heart rate going will suffice.

What can I do about my current posture?

Address and consistently practice these considerations of posture as early as possible. Many of my patients, after doing yoga for six or seven months without evident improvement in their posture, ask why they see little improvement. I always answer that if it's taken them a lifetime to achieve inadequate posture, it will surely take them several years to overcome it. And it will take daily, or at least two to three times weekly, exercise sessions to lengthen the muscles, impart flexibility to the joints affected by those muscles, so as to lengthen the tendons and ligaments and slowly gain the flexibility and healthy posture of a teenager. You need time and patience; many of you are now paying the price for addressing cardiovascular fitness at the expense of musculoskeletal health.

How shall I start?

The first step in rehabilitating posture is to determine and address any defects such as a shorter leg or scoliosis. For example, can you balance and correct that shorter leg with a shoe insert? Once such minor defects are corrected, you can begin stretching your muscles. If the defect is scoliosis, for instance, and cannot be corrected, then certain exercises emphasizing the loosening of tighter areas constitute appropriate preparation for further stretching. It may take some time to make your muscles flexible enough, that is to have a range of motion great enough, to move forward. Eventually, however, you will be able to achieve healthier posture.

Women, look to the dancer—not the ballerina but the modern dancer—for a model. Dancers have extremely flexible, lean and long, powerful muscles with good definition. They are lively and graceful in motion.

Men, look to Cirque du Soleil performers, who move with surprising agility and flexibility. These men are muscular and tremendously strong. Forget the football players, most of whom are far too stiff to have good range of motion. They do have bursts of energy, but they do not have enough flexibility to prevent injury. Body builders are in the same category. Watch any man carrying a six-pack in his abdomen—usually his shoulders are sloped and hunched over, his abdominal muscles pulling his upper body forward. A flexible abdominalis is better than a tight one. You want the external oblique to be strong, pulling your tummy in—not a tight abdominalis pulling the shoulder forward and compressing your spine.

Is there anything besides exercise that will help?

Achieving hormone balance may be important to restoring muscle health. Growth hormone, for example, has been known to prevent older people from losing muscle mass. Hormones like DHEA, testosterone, and related types also have been shown to preserve musculature in elders. Vigorous exercise releases some of these hormones from the pituitary gland in the brain. Supplementing these hormones is controversial; choose to follow such a course only with the help of your physician.

We know that IGF-1, an indicator of growth hormone from the insulin family, must reside within the muscle cells for the muscles to grow. And the hormone myostatin limits the growth of muscles by breaking muscles into finer components. IGF-1 and myostatin must be in balance to maintain muscle integrity. As one ages, one tends to lose this balance, gradually lose muscle, and become thinner. Again, exercise helps preserve muscle mass, so in addition to hormone balance, you need constant stretching work and a thoughtful, balanced choice of strengthening exercise for maximum health.

Remember, finally, to stretch the cervical neck and shoulder muscles of the shoulder girdle—the scalene bundles that, unless they are flexible, will pull your neck forward and exacerbate compression. Exercise the quadratus lumborum and psoas on the lower back and the gluteus and piriformis muscles on the lower rump. Joseph Pilates, creator of the now popular Pilates exercise, often says, "You are as old as the flexibility of your spine." The less flexible your spine, the older you look, and the more flexible your spine, the younger you look. More important, if you remain flexible, you will retain musculoskeletal health for a much longer period of time.

What about Bones? A New Look at Osteoporosis

I've noticed that many friends of my age—friends who are healthy and live vital lives—are beginning to notice their borderline status in bone-density tests.

Bones provide the framework for the body, literally holding its health together. And aging bones are threatened by osteoporosis—a 21st-century epidemic, a silent disease undetectable without a bone-density scan. Americans are ingesting more than

12 million prescriptions for "bone-building" drugs annually, but those prescriptions are not doing the job. Neither are calcium supplements.

I have paid attention to my bone-mass tests for years, thinking a "normal" result (that of the average woman of my age) is not good enough. After all, as noted earlier, bone mass begins to decrease at age 35, then continues downward. I do not want to be normal but to be optimal—15 to 20 percent above normal. That is the goal my sister and I set out to achieve, and so far we've been successful.

We began with our brother, Dr. Sam Yue, to find out what is possible, to read and learn what can be done. One article in *O, The Oprah Magazine* told how Rose Kushner and Janine O'Leary convinced doctors to change their protocols (see pages 74 and 170). It reminded me that we must be our own health activists. I don't want to wait years for doctors to run into a disaster such as the Premarin® problem before finding their recommendations have been wrong. I believe in the old art of medicine—observing many patients, learning about what is important and what works, and validating conclusions with exhaustive research.

The Great Pharmacopoeia by Li Shi-zhen is an example of how someone tried to put it all together in that way. Four centuries ago he spent 30 years traveling the countryside of China, gathering information from local doctors, documenting diseases, and cross-referencing them with plants and herbs effective in treating people and animals. His book is still used today in Traditional Chinese Medicine (TCM). Right now China teaches both Eastern and Western medicine to budding physicians. My cousin, studying for a Western medical degree in China, spent 30 percent of her time studying TCM.

Let me share with you how I have come to preserve my own bone health.

Most experts mention only half the equation—bone mass/calcium—and not collagen, which is just as important in forming healthy bone. I have arrived at this conclusion partly through my brother's observation of his patients using relaxin in his pain clinic. Alternative therapists such as chiropractor David Williams have done a good job of helping us to understand the importance of keeping the body in an alkaline state so as to absorb calcium. But they mention little about the hormone balance important to healthy collagen for bone growth. If you solve only one piece of the puzzle, you still have a puzzle. And collagen is the missing link!

First, we tackled calcium absorption. Of all I've read, I highly recommend David Williams's special report *Better Bone-Builder and More Lifesavers for Women.* Second, we learned through my brother's treatment of FMS patients. Third, we read more, eventually finding a study by William H. Parker, M.D., and his colleagues involving 10,000 women with ovaries removed who suffered an additional 157 deaths related to hip fractures. Putting together the information from all these sources, we came up with a new concept—that the three major hormones produced by the ovaries—estrogen, progesterone, and relaxin, the Cinderella hormone—play a big part in the health of aging bones. (Sam will tell you about that later.)

First, what can we do naturally for our bones? Eat right.

David Williams, D.C., and most alternative therapists, agree that maintaining a pH level more alkaline than acid is best. The ideal level is pH 7.4 When pH drops below that, even to 7.38, the body becomes acidic enough to break down bone and muscle tissues—so as to use their alkalizing ammonia, carbonates, and phosphates. In addition to supporting the body, the bones serve as the body's storage facility for acid-neutralizing minerals. Anthony Sebastian and Deborah Sellmeyer at the University of California reviewed more than 85 studies from 33 countries, discovering a direct relationship between diets high in animal protein (such as fish, meat, and cheese) and the incidence of hip fracture. Germany and Sweden, with high consumption of these foods, showed 40 times more hip fractures than did Thailand. The Thai people eat a lot more vegetables and fruits.

How to Maintain Alkaline pH

The most important factor is what you eat. Studies show that women athletes eating five to six servings of fruits and vegetables compared to those eating fewer than three servings evidence lower levels of calcium in their urine. That confirms the theory of bones storing acid-neutralizing minerals.

The body's storage of calcium is in a constant state of transformation, or "bone remodeling," with the bones acting as a storehouse for calcium reserves. Roughly 99 percent of the body's total calcium is in bones and teeth, the other 1 percent in body fluids and soft tissue. Calcium is drawn from the bones when blood and tissue levels are too low. Any excesses of calcium are deposited in the bones. Research shows that under normal circumstances the calcium in bones is replaced about every ten years.

Dietary surveys have revealed that the levels of calcium in bone decrease as the phosphorus levels in food rise and calcium becomes insufficient to reverse the trend. So, the *Tao of Youth* eating strategy discussed in Key 1 is good for bone health—eating lots of fruit and vegetables puts your body in a more alkaline state. So you can kill two birds with one stone—lose water weight as you build healthy bone!

High Calcium

Certain nutrients like calcium, iron, and protein require high hydrochloric acid levels in the stomach to digest properly. By age 50, the stomach releases only 15 percent of the amount released at age 25. And 35 percent of those past age 65 do not produce hydrochloric acid at all. According to Dr. Williams, this explains why calcium deficiencies often occur in older patients, along with high blood pressure, heart palpitations, tremors, osteoporosis, insomnia, leg cramps, nervousness, and irritability.

So, yes, we need to ingest enough calcium, but it won't do any good if it's not absorbed. In selecting a calcium supplement, look for one that contains betaine hydrochloride, additional magnesium, and vitamin D. My brother Sam recommends chelated calcium for better absorption.

Low Phosphorus

Phosphorus is a mineral important to good health, but an excess of phosphorus can lead to serious problems. More than 45 different phosphorus-containing chemicals are added to foods—especially to frozen pizza, chicken, and fish—as preservatives of color and moisture and as emulsifiers and sequestrates. Additionally, more than 70 phosphorus compounds become indirect additives from packaging materials, sanitizers, and production acids (see David Williams's special report).

Eating a high-phosphorus diet, especially if you are low in calcium, leads to osteoporosis. With the high increase of phosphorus in foods during the last decade, no wonder we have so many bone problems. So, readjust your phosphorus/calcium levels by cutting your intake of soft drinks, and integrate a wider variety of fresh foods into your diet. Processed and frozen food dishes are loaded with phosphorus and phosphate not even listed on food labels. You cannot go wrong if you go back to the ancients—they ate something very close to the *Tao of Youth* food regimen.

Sweet Xylitol

Researchers in Finland have been working on a natural sweetener for 25 years. Xylitol is a compound found naturally in strawberries, raspberries, plums, and jute as well as in hardwood trees like birch. When used as a sweetener in chewing gum, xylitol is a powerful tool for preventing dental cavities and plaque formation.

Finnish animal studies suggest that xylitol helps maintain and even increase bone density. I recommend using xylitol instead of sugar made of sucrose.

Hormone Balance—A New Idea about Bones

There is a definite relationship between the balance of hormones and the health of bones. My brother Sam is the world's expert when it comes to clinical observations on the use of relaxin for healthy collagen and bone. Here's what he told me:

Osteoporosis is a common problem in the United States and in developing countries in the Western hemisphere. It is extremely common among fibromyalgia patients, who age faster than the normal population. Their experience provides a sort of preview for the normally aging adult.

What do you first see in fibromyalgia patients that suggests they have osteoporosis? And what are the risk factors for this disease?

Osteoporosis commonly presents degeneration in the joints of fibromyalgia patients. Extreme stress on the joints because of tight and spastic muscles and ligaments results in further degeneration. Still, osteoporosis in fibromyalgia patients, and probably in the aging general population, is due mainly to poor collagen.

While there are many risk factors for osteoporosis, one factor commonly mentioned but rarely addressed is the quality of collagen in the bone matrix (the generator of bone). The integrity of bone depends on two things: the quality of the collagen and the amount of calcium. A deficit in either one results in osteoporosis.

The congenital disease called osteogenic imperfection, or brittle bones, for example, is the result of collagen defect. Even minor stress to brittle bones causes fracture, even to fetuses inside their mothers' wombs. But these young patients' bones are extremely dense. The broken bones heal quickly, almost immediately, due to dense deposits of calcium within the fractures. It's not a lack of calcium—but the lack of quality collagen—that causes their bones to break easily.

So two elements determine the makeup of healthy bones, but most healthcare providers focus on calcium and tend to ignore the quality of the collagen. Testing for bone health, for instance, consists of measuring bone density—determining the amount of calcium or determining what and how the bone structure handles calcium. Such measurement ignores the quality of collagen in the bony matrix, which allows the bone to hold onto calcium, which lends the bone its tensile strength.

Can you make that less complicated?

Healthy bone has elements similar to the cement and iron rods of a building—the iron rod is the calcium and the collagen is the cement. Even good cement (collagen) cannot hold up a building without enough iron rods (the calcium). Likewise, even many iron rods cannot prevent the walls of a building from breaking if the cement (the collagen) is poor. Calcium and healthy collagen are equally important.

What makes for good collagen? Why does estrogen and progesterone replacement (HRT) in menopausal women not restore enough calcium?

I believe that collagen degenerates quickly in most menopausal women and that the phenomenon is related not to deficits of estrogen or progesterone but to a deficit of relaxin. Relaxin directly governs the collagen structure in the bony matrix, giving rise to a good quality of collagen, resulting in better-quality bone that holds onto calcium and thus is stronger. Even with smaller amounts of calcium, if the collagen is good, the bone will be more resilient, elastic, and less likely to fracture.

Is there research showing this?

Sure. The people in Germany and Sweden, who consume large amounts of calcium-rich milk, meat, and protein, have been shown to have a high incidence of hip fracture as opposed to those in Thailand who consume less meat and milk. The pH balance (the Thai diet is heavily alkaline and the German and Swedish diets are heavily acidic) also plays a role in calcium deposits, but the quality of the bone affected by the quality of collagen is equally important.

There are no tests for measuring the role that deficits of relaxin play in the osteoporosis of artificially or naturally induced menopausal women. While calcium, vitamin D, other hormonal deficits, and other factors may play some role, they do not wholly explain the incidence of osteoporosis in developed countries of the Western world. Perhaps relaxin plays a bigger role than all the other factors combined.

So you think relaxin may be even more important than calcium?

Of the two deficits leading to osteoporosis, I believe the more important is the quality of the bony matrix as related to the activity of relaxin on collagen. I strongly suggest women take relaxin for a better quality of collagen. I also recommend that women pay attention to both conventional and alternative medicine approaches to bone health. Calcium, natural progesterone, and estrogen supplements may play a role in increasing calcium absorption and the quality of the bony matrix. Medications inhibiting the absorption of calcium may also play a role. But pH balance is key, and alternative medicine addresses this balance better than conventional medicine.

What difference does pH balance make?

Briefly, pH affects the formation and reabsorption of calcium within the bone as well as the absorption of calcium in the GI (gastrointestinal) tract. Studies indicate that young, healthy, athletic women who consume less than three servings of fruits and vegetables excrete calcium in their urine. Women who consume more than three servings of fruits and vegetables do not excrete calcium. (You can Google other sources on this subject—many alternative physicians give detailed explanations of how and why pH and other factors affect the bone health of older women and men.) From this result, one might infer the following:

The Western diet includes too much acid-forming food, impacting pH balance—that is, making the body acidic—when it operates best with a slightly alkaline balance. When the body is acidic, it tends to break down or leach many of the alkaline minerals (including calcium) from bone and other tissues as well as to secrete bile and other enzymes to neutralize the acidity.

Let's focus on the calcium here. In the process of neutralizing acidity, calcium leached from the bone enters the blood. Because of the higher level of calcium in the blood, the kidneys excrete calcium to bring the level back to normal, which in turn causes the bone to leach more calcium into the blood—again to neutralize acidity. So, when you eat a constantly acidic diet, the body gradually leaches calcium, slowly excreting some of it in urine. At the same time the high level of calcium in the blood keeps the gut from absorbing calcium. Most of the consumed calcium, then, passes through the GI tract without being absorbed, in a vicious cycle.

So taking more calcium doesn't solve the problem?

We know that daily calcium supplements are not easily absorbed unless the blood contains a lower level of calcium than is normal. To reverse the process, the blood level of calcium must drop to balance acidity with alkalinity. Calcium then is absorbed—from the GI tract into the blood to achieve the normal level—and transported back to build stronger bones.

For good balance you must eat in a way that slowly changes pH from an acidic to a slightly alkaline balance. This requires eating 80 percent alkaline-forming and 20 percent acid-forming foods. Or *eat 80 percent fruits and vegetables and 20 percent everything else.* Most fruits and vegetables are alkaline-forming, and most meats, grains, and processed food and sugars are acid-forming. Many other books describe the best ways of eating to minimize acidity.

Do medications such as Fosamax® make a difference?

They inhibit the breakdown and absorption of old bone into the body but do not contribute to the formation of new bone. In a healthy individual, old bone breaks down and new bone forms in a balanced cycle. Prohibiting the absorption of old bone allows more calcium to remain, but that does not on its own produce good-quality bone. Without addressing the issue of pH and the deposit of calcium necessary for new bone formation, Fosamax® increases bone density through increasing the quantity of calcium but does not address the quality of the bone—that is, its formation from a bony matrix containing high-quality collagen that holds onto the calcium necessary for healthy bone. Again, the health of the bone depends on two elements—calcium and high-quality collagen. Together they form strong, healthy bones, and together they prevent age-related osteoporosis.

What are some visible signs of osteoporosis? How will I know if I have it?

One visible sign of osteoporosis is the loss of teeth. Few pay much attention to the relationship between the health of the bones and the teeth. Many fibromyalgia (male and female) patients lose teeth earlier than the healthy population, for two reasons: (1) calcium erodes in the teeth (osteoporosis), and (2) the bony sockets of the jaw do not hold teeth firmly because osteodegenerative changes occur in both the sockets and the teeth. Few people realize that teeth are part of the bony structure and that the sockets of the teeth within the facial bones are joints. So losing teeth in your forties or fifties is an early indication of the development of osteoporosis. X-rays and bone density tests also reveal early indicators for osteoporosis.

Are there further indications that collagen is important to bone development?

Osteopenic (borderline osteoporosis) patients with good-quality bone matrix do not fracture as easily as nonosteopenic patients with higher bone density but poor-quality collagen. In fact, those with poor collagen break their bones much more easily. For instance, diabetic patients, who usually have poorer-quality collagen, have a higher incidence of fracture than the normal population. Further, the posture of these patients often reveals signs of osteoporosis. Posture is usually exaggerated in those with a strong history of osteoporosis within their immediate families.

I'm pretty healthy. What do you recommend I do to prevent osteoporosis?

The bottom line is my suggestion that, if you are aware of severe osteoporosis in close family members, you take relaxin in the form of Biolaxin™ once in the morning and once at bedtime, as well as calcium (chelated calcium, which is easily absorbed and does not upset the stomach) and other anti-osteoporosis supplements. Take 180 mg of chelated calcium and 100 mg of chelated magnesium together two to three times a day. And get as close to eating 80 percent fruits and vegetables as you can!

Alternative medicine authorities such as David Williams, D.C., Susan Lark, M.D., and Julian Whitaker, M.D., have addressed other factors, including the benefits of phosphorus calcium, to good effect. The point here is that pH balance, achieved through a slightly more alkaline than acidic diet, plus the retention of quality collagen and thus calcium, plays a huge part in the health of your bones and teeth.

Coming Around

Just as I began the conclusion of this section, my brother Sam found an article in *New York Times* titled "To Avoid 'Boomeritis.' Exercise, Exercise, Exercise." The story reiterates most of the concepts observed by Sam through his pain practice and described above. Dr. Sam has always maintained that beyond walking, jogging, cycling, and swimming to promote endurance, cardiovascular health, and weight control, there is a great need for exercise to improve posture and increase flexibility and balance, and then strength. Such exercise greatly reduces the risk of injury from sports and the demands of daily life, from falls and other accidents.

I have noticed that some fitness experts are beginning to say the same things. We baby boomers are developing tendonitis, bursitis, arthritis, and other related muscle problems. To counter the inevitable decline of age, we must provide our bodies an extended warranty. The kind of exercise I've been doing is meant to do just that. Bikram yoga and Pilates routines provide flexibility, posture, strength, and balance.

Recently my sister Cathy and I took up belly dancing to round out our exercise routines. Belly dancing works on muscles in the hip and abdominal regions that we had never used before and adds strength to legs and arms (you have to raise your arms a lot when you belly dance).

I have no talent and no intention of subjecting others to my belly dancing as performance, but I enjoy the classes and laugh a lot in every one. And my yoga instructor has noticed improvement in my yoga practice since I started belly dancing.

The idea is to do exercise that works on your weak muscles as well as building your core strength. As we age, we must include flexibility in our exercise regimens—then strength and balance. Otherwise, strength will decline as muscle fibers decrease in size and number and as nerve stimulation and energy to the muscles diminish. Balance also deteriorates as muscles tighten and weaken and joints lose their full range of motion. Flexibility declines as connective tissue throughout the body becomes less elastic, and endurance decreases with reduced flexibility, weakened muscles, and stiffer lungs and blood vessels. My brother Sam has strong ideas about how to keep bone mass in good shape as presented earlier.

As to the notion of Tao in our approach to musculoskeletal wellness—harmony and balance, yin and yang, are the watchwords. One thing I cannot emphasize enough is that you take from our findings what is best for you, ask your own questions, and build on the answers. I chose a Botox® injection in my piriformis muscle, an invasive process to numb pain so that I could rehab other muscles and get back to normal. It worked for me—now all the muscles around my hip areas are flexible—but such a thing might not be your cup of tea. It makes sense to take advantage of new information and technology as well as ancient knowledge to accomplish your physical fitness.

We cannot wait for the medical community to give us right answers. We must be our own advocates for good muscles, bones, and teeth. Key 3—the way to healthy musculoskeletal structure—is an important part of the *Tao of Youth*. You cannot live an active, vital life if you cannot get around. You cannot afford to compromise your mobility with a hip fracture. Key 3 is a prescription for balance, one in which bone and muscle go hand in hand.

Choose the strategy best for you. We are born with differing asymmetries and different personalities and tolerances. Customize an exercise regimen to achieve musculoskeletal health in ways you are likely to follow through. Tao is a path, your path to harmony and balance. Maintaining good physical fitness as you age will enable you to participate comfortably in a greater variety activities, giving you greater freedom, independence, and joy.

Key 4

Understanding the whole you:

Unifying mind, body, spirit

My Journey towards Three-part Being

What do we mean by the integration of mind, body, and spirit? Such integration is the evolution into a higher level of understanding, bringing bodily desires into balance with mind and soul. We are three-part beings—made of body, mind, and soul—but most of us experience ourselves only as physical bodies. We feed our bodies, clothe them, get some sleep. We live as one-part beings, often not doing a good job even of that.

Many of us do not read any more; at least, we don't read books from which we can learn something. We do not nourish our minds intellectually. We become dull. We do not ask questions. We are not really awake. And our minds do not expand.

As we age, we tend to disengage our minds even more. And we don't feed them well in a physical way—many people cling to the idea that if they eat good food they are well nourished. They don't ask about the soil the food grows in, for instance, about whether the soil has been depleted of nutrients. In truth, because we are in such a hurry to produce the most crops in the shortest time, we have ruined much of the soil in this country. Ask every question you can think of about what is good for you. Use your mind.

Even those few who do honor the mind and body use no more than one-tenth of their brain's capacity. If you knew what your mind is capable of, you would never cease to wonder at its power.

We are three-part beings. We are more than body, and we are more than body and mind. Do we notice and nurture the soul? Do we even think about it? Are we healing or hurting it? When was the last time you expressed your soul? Listened to those whispered longings buried deep inside? When was the last time your cried with joy, acted silly, wrote poetry, danced in the nude, kissed a baby, sang in the rain, painted a picture, gazed at a rainbow, communed with nature, searched for God?

When was the last time you sat alone with the silence to travel to the deepest part of your being, said hello to your soul? Or the last time you looked into a mirror and said, "I love my soul," acknowledging your beautiful spirit?

Living as single-part persons, we become deeply mired in matters of the body: money, sex, power, possessions, physical stimulation and satisfaction, security, fame, financial gain. As dual-part persons, we also recognize matters of the mind: creativity, the stimulation of new ideas and thoughts, goals, challenges, and personal growth.

But as three-part persons, we come into balance, concerned with matters of the soul as well: spiritual identity, life purpose, relationship to God, evolution, spiritual growth, destiny. Evolving into higher states of consciousness, we realize new aspects of being. This does not mean dropping one part of the self in favor of others. It simply means expanding one's focus, turning away from exclusive involvement with one aspect, towards love and appreciation of all.

As a girl I saw cute "little old ladies" with pink cheeks and melting smiles. Thinking of them, I eventually had a revelation: "They have achieved something—that is what is needed in that beauty-cream jar." Now I believe that beautiful older women have integrated all aspects of their being. Their faces tell me they are truly satisfied.

The five keys of the *Tao of Youth* show you the path we have taken and the tools we have discovered along the way—tools that may help you to achieve the integration of the three facets of your being. I have found that feeding my body and stimulating my mind are not enough—I must also nourish my soul. The music offered here has helped me to pursue that aspect of my life without fear. And I know that when I nourish my soul, it shows in my face and body, in fact in every aspect of my life.

I first started questioning my life when I visited my homeland at age 37. I left China when I was four years old and was going back there to visit after 33 years (China closed the border after 1950).

My aunt once looked at me and said, "You and your sisters were like two little urchins squatting on the ground, waiting for the ferry to leave for Hong Kong like refugees." She said her heart was aching because she had no idea what our fate would be. "You could drown or be injured by the bombing from Taiwan or even be taken to Taiwan. The trip was treacherous, yet your parents had chosen this route." She and her husband had decided to stay put in Xiamen.

Ours was the last ferry to leave Xiamen and reach Hong Kong—for 30 years. China was at war (the regimes of Mao and Chiang Kai Shek). Our relatives fled to different parts of China, and some had gone to the U.S.A. The ferry following ours was bombed. Our landing in Hong Kong determined our fate, one very different from that of our aunts and cousins. We were not able to see them over all that time.

I was the first of my family in the West to visit China and see my relatives there. My late, favorite business partner said when I was leaving, "May, this trip to China will define your life." She was right. I wish she could see what I am doing now.

At the time I visited, China was just opening up. Contact with the Western world was still limited, but I saw inklings of progress. My cousins, whom I had never met because they were born after I left China, had lived through a lot of hardship; because of our family background, the government had not allowed them to attend school. One of my cousins, whom later I sponsored to come to the United States for a law degree, had taught herself English and was teaching English at the University of Xiamen.

The spirit of our family's need to achieve had lived on in the face of suppression. One of my male cousins became a well-known dancer in Fujian. He had represented my hometown in performances in Beijing, but he came back to Xiamen to see the first visitor from our family in the West in 33 years. The meal he hosted for my then-husband and me cost him a year's salary.

Everything in China was new to me because I had not been there since I was a child. Because I was traveling with the Minnesota Trade Commission, I attended some banquets with officials as well as visiting my relatives and doing some sightseeing. I was absorbing all the new sights, sounds, food, and odors and getting to know so many new faces at the same time.

My relatives treated me like the most honored guest, and everyone—about 30 relatives including some only distantly related—came to see me. My mother had instructed me to give each of them some money—my family had been supporting many of our relatives there for 33 years, from Hong Kong. Chinese families stick together. Today they are all doing well and do not require our support.

I was in China only three days before we were to leave by plane to go back to Hong Kong. But then we were told we could not take the plane because my husband was an American, and no American could be allowed in the air as he might determine landmarks. So we took the overnight ferry back to Hong Kong. On the ferry, I realized I was reliving the trip of my childhood to Hong Kong from Xiamen. The ferry was of typical Chinese style—its interior decorated with a gaudy red, though it was not in any way a luxurious boat. I was not too happy with the accommodations, but I knew that just one night would pass before we arrived in Hong Kong.

During the crossing, we decided to go up to the deck—it was winter, so no one else was there. The swimming pool on the upper deck was lined with Spanish tiles! As later came to light, the vessel was an old Portuguese ferry. The Chinese government's partial renovation had certainly left something to be desired.

I came back into the cabin, and for some reason I looked into the mirror and said, "I am like this boat—a funny mix. Who am I? I am neither Chinese nor American. I look as ridiculous as this ferry."

My cousins had had a lot less to work with, yet they had achieved a lot. I had had many more opportunities and felt at the time that I was not using all that was given to me compared to what my cousins had done. They had an identity, and I did not.

That ferry trip, during which I relived my experience as a four-year-old, was a defining moment. From that day on I committed myself to defining my unifying principles and living in accord with them. Little did I know when I began that journey that I had started on a path that would change the shape of my life.

Neither did I know that in plowing this path I would have to make many painful decisions or that this was the beginning of my spiritual journey.

Upon my return, like many people, I began to read transformation and self-help books. I started a ritual—whenever I am in a bookstore I let my feelings guide me to choosing the next book to read. The book *Return to Love* by Marianne Williamson just stared at me when I went into the bookstore after my return from that first trip back to China. I still use that method to choose books. I do not read any critic's choice but use my feelings to decide. As a result I have read my share of New Age literature—all of Shirley MacLaine's books and all of Williamson's, too. I also read biographies, as I like to know what makes people tick. I have read all of the Dalai Lama's books, thinking that if he was the world's most gifted guru, I would like them, and I did.

In all these books I have found wisdom related to the painful events in my life, some of them the result of decisions related to taking my new path. I have gone through much "humble time," developing an understanding of how to deal with my pain, realizing how self-centered I was, beginning to feel empathy for others. It took a lot of reading and thinking to reach an understanding of myself and to come to know what I want. Finally, I started to live my life with joy.

I have not yet mastered all the skills I need to conduct my life joyfully. I can only say that I have come a long way and that I feel so much more at peace with myself than I did before.

So what have I learned on this journey, and how can it help you?

I read that the Dalai Lama gets up every morning to chant for a couple hours. He does it every day and finds great joy in the practice. I read many books too of gurus such as Osho and other yogis. Just about all of them tell us to meditate to achieve nirvana. Reading further, I found a study noting that when a harmonious Buddhist monks' community stopped chanting and meditating for three months, its members argued and fought. When their chanting and meditation resumed, they became happy and harmonious again.

When I read that I thought, "I want to do this meditation and chanting." I found the Tibetan Quan Yin chant—"om mani pad me hom." I start practicing it but found I had a hard time getting into it, until one day I met Gary Hovda. He produces a certain kind of music, and I found that when I listen to it, I get into the Quan Yin chant right away. The ancients discovered the frequencies of chanting that caused their bodies to vibrate to a good state. Gary's music produced that state in a much shorter time. Instant meditation!

Given our busy lives, finding a way to reach a meditative state without chanting for two hours is a blessing, one I would like to share. Read my interview with Gary; then enjoy the CD included with this book. Without doing anything active, you can take your first step on the path of the *Tao of Youth*. Just put it into your CD player or load it onto your iPod, and listen. The vibration and frequency of this music may replicate in you the alpha state of the monks I visited in a Tibetan monastery in Yunan Province.

How I Learned about the *Tao of Music*

I met Gary Hovda through a mutual friend. A week later Gary invited us to come to a beautiful house he had designed—to listen to music he had developed.

Gary had asked a few other people to join us for the event. An active, eight-year-old girl was there with her mother and friends. I noticed that she ran into the bathroom, jumped into the tub, and curled up there. She did not make any eye contact or acknowledge me in any way, even though I was the only one in the bathroom with her (I was taking a tour of the house at the time).

After the house tour, we all went into the media room. A DVD player displayed a bluish oval image on a screen accompanied by subcellular music. The minute I walked into the room I noticed a vibration in my throat chakra area. I felt a little strange; I did not usually respond to music in that way. The music seemed to follow the wall around the room. That's when I noticed that the room was not oval as I had thought, but that it had an elliptical shape.

Gary told us how he produced the music—that one night when he played it outside in a field on a mountaintop in the state of Washington, he had noticed a lot of energy bubbles such as he had felt with the same frequency in the pyramids in Egypt. (Sometime you can see energy bubbles when you flash a digital camera. I have experienced that kind of energy in the landscape of Yunan.) Gary discovered this elliptical shape in a photo that a friend took of him while playing the music on the mountaintop. This was the image playing on the screen in his media room.

Then I noticed the little girl I had met in the bathroom, lying against her mother in a comfortable, open-armed position, the way my dog Yoko does when she feels safe and lets her tummy hang out. This child, Annie, obviously felt safe and calm. She asked, "When you are up in the mountains at night, aren't you afraid of the wild animals?" Charmed by her curiosity, I responded by walking over to her, and we carried on a lively conversation.

After some time in the media room, I felt the music was a bit too much for me and walked to another part of the house. But when I came back, I became used to it and enjoyed it, and Gary gave me a CD as we left the house. I immediately put it into my car player and turned it on. I felt relaxed, my brain clear. I was able to solve a problem I had been thinking about, and I felt great relief on doing so.

At the time I had been trying to use the Quan Yin chant for meditation—with little success. I decided to play Gary's music and see what happened. I found that the music and the chant vibrated in similar ways, making it easy for me to sink into the chant. I immediately called Gary to tell him what had happened.

Later I found out that the girl I had met at Gary's house is autistic. Rarely did she interact with strangers, yet at Gary's client's house with the music playing she had become comfortable enough to carry on a conversation. Gary told me that her parents were delighted with exposure to the music she was slowly opening and beginning to participate in many of the activities around her. Soon after the gathering in the media room, I attended a regular meeting of the board of the National Association for International Educators (NAFSA) in Washington, DC. After these meetings, we usually went to the executive director's home for dinner. I asked whether I could play Gary's music so the people there would be more relaxed, and our host agreed.

The music had just started, and I was still at the CD player when a board member dashed over to ask about the music.

"What is that?" she asked, her eyes wide. Her intensity startled me.

She sat next to the CD player, tears streaming down her cheeks. I didn't know what to do—I thought I had done something wrong and offered to stop it.

"No! No! Leave it on," she said. "I've had this headache all day long and I have tinnitus. I always have a ringing sound in my ears. It was so bad today—then the music just released the tension. And that's why the tears started to fall."

I promised that when I got home I would send her the CD. I was amazed at the power of the musical vibration; apparently it neutralized the ringing in her ears.

About a month later, a childhood friend of mine was dying, and I received a call from his cousin as to his deteriorating condition. I spoke to my friend, saying I would fly to Hong Kong to see him. His family thought I would be too late, but I knew he would wait for me.

My friend was still alive when I walked into the hospital room with his cousin. I saw his pain-filled face, his three children crying. When he saw me, a tear rolled down his cheek. I immediately asked one of the nurses to find a CD player, then turned on the CD of Gary's music, putting the earphone into my friend's ear. I asked his children and his cousin to massage him and talk to him. We laughed and talked and lived in that moment. He became more relaxed; a peace came over his face. Five hours later he died in total peace..

One of his daughters thanked his cousin and me for coming. She had not seen that peacefulness earlier, and she believed the difference was in the music. I gave her the CD. And I now give this music to you as a gift because it brings so much joy and peacefulness to me. (Find a CD with a sample of Gary's music in the back.)

If stress is a factor in early aging (and studies indicate it is), this music that relieves stress can help you to ease quickly into a restful state, what is referred to as an alpha state. As part of the *Tao of Youth*, it simply makes sense for me so share this discovery.

As a result of this music, I have noticed a new ease, for instance, in writing this book. I just turn on the music—sometimes I meditate with the music on my iPod in my garden in front of 16 round stones arranged exactly in the shape of the blue orb playing on the screen in Gary's client's house. He helped me put that together after discovering that the shape has the same mathematical frequency as the music.

I'll let Gary tell you about how he found this key to peace, harmony, and serenity. Suffice it for now to say that the music and elliptical shape provide a frequency and vibration that resonate with humans to the extent that they ease one into an alpha state—where the mind, body, and spirit are in synchrony and so perform at their best. Everyone exposed to this music seems to feel its positive effects right away.

Peace Begins at the Cellular Level—How Cellusonic Music Works

Cellusonic music has proved a boon to my life—an increasing peace and calmness and a pulling together of the power of my brain. For a long time, probably like you, I have understood that certain vitamins and minerals could help my brain, but I had certainly never thought that music could make me "smarter." Here's Gary's explanation of how the power of music can relieve stress and nourish your brain. Stress is a well-known cause of early aging, so this is a powerful tool for maintaining your equilibrium and good health.

Gary, what can this music do for me?

Have you ever heard that human beings use only 10 percent of their potential brainpower and wondered why? Or why nearly 19 million Americans are diagnosed with depression each year? Many intellectual, psychic, and emotional problems are linked to disturbances in the natural frequencies that exist both in our bodies and in the natural world around us. Cellusonic music may help.

The copyrighted cellusonic music included with this book impacts the brain by tuning it into frequencies found in nature. The brain naturally resonates with these frequencies, and the benefits are quick and dramatic. Cellusonic music:

- relieves your stress and anxiety
- optimizes your concentration, focus, and ability to learn
- improves your memory
- expands your creativity
- increases your motivation and boosts your confidence
- provides a sense of "infinite time" and gradual spiritual awakening
- promotes better chi (energy) in your internal organs
- contributes to your overall mental, spiritual, and physical health.

Inner peace and an improved brain state don't have to cost thousands of dollars or years of practice. We'd all like to be able to devote several hours a day to meditation to improve our mental and spiritual health. But most of us are far too busy to follow such a time-consuming personal-growth program. Cellusonic music uses science to help you obtain your personal-growth goals without complicated regimens or unnecessary expense.

How does cellusonic music work?

Certain types of music lend themselves to relaxation and thus allow the skin and body to absorb nutrients in an efficient way. Physicians Andrew Weil and Jonathan Wright have written about the benefits of music compatible with alpha brainwaves (those of a brain in a resting state). The concept is not new, but using it as part of a body-and-mind wellness program is revolutionary.

The *Tao of Youth* alpha-wave-compatible music offers powerful healing qualities because its sound is based on frequencies found in nature and in the brain's natural resting state. As the brain recognizes alpha waves, it begins to resonate along the same frequencies, much like a tuning fork. This allows listeners to relax and bring their brains into a state not unlike that of a chanting Tibetan monk. At the same time it reduces electrical skin resistance to a level facilitating the absorption of enzymes and of therapeutic formulations applied to the skin.

This music—let's call it the *Tao of Music*—allows for optimum absorption, for instance, of the *Tao of Youth* Biolaxin™ (relaxin) skin cream and of the Biolaxin™ (relaxin) food supplement.

What is a brainwave? Are there different kinds?

Your brain is made up of nerves that constantly generate electrical impulses called brainwave patterns. These patterns make up your thoughts, emotions, and state of being, and they determine the level of functioning of various systems of your body.

Brainwaves occur in four distinct patterns and have been assigned names from the Greek alphabet:

- Delta brainwaves occur while a person is asleep or unconscious.
- Theta brainwaves occur during sleep and have been linked to the state of dreaming—the "REM" state of sleep accompanied by rapid eye movement.
- Beta brainwaves occur when a person is alert and aware of the happenings in the world around them.
- Alpha brainwaves occur when a person is awake but in a relaxed, passive state of mind, in a state of well-being, or meditation.

When your brain is in normal waking consciousness, it emits a beta-wave pattern. Beta waves indicate concentration, arousal, alertness, and cognition. At a heightened state, beta waves may mean anxiety, disharmony, and discord. A stressful day is one full of beta waves.

When you are at ease, your brain emits an alpha-wave pattern. Alpha patterns are associated with relaxation, super-learning, increased serotonin levels (fending off depression), meditation, and the beginning of access to your subconscious mind. Chanting monks reside in the deepest state of alpha—a more focused but still relaxed state. The *Tao of Music* promotes this brain state and increases your concentration and ability to learn.

How does this cellusonic music work as part of the *Tao of Youth*?

Listening to cellusonic music for 10 minutes at least once a day is an essential element of the *Tao of Youth*. The *Tao of Music* helps to promote physical and mental health at the cellular level through sonic vibrations, making the body more easily able to absorb helpful enzymes and food supplements for the body's youthful inner balance as well as appropriate topical skin therapies.

The scientific community widely recognizes that certain degrees of emotional stress change the physiological state of the skin. This is scientifically referred to as galvanic skin response (see page 125). Due mainly to emotional stress, electrical resistance in the skin may limit or counteract the therapeutic effectiveness of lotions or biological formulations that could otherwise assist in healing/rejuvenation. Such resistance is affected not only by the subject's general mood but also by the subject's immediate reaction to a stimulus.

Although Jean de Tarchanoff first wrote about the Tarchanoff, or galvanic, response in 1890, the underlying causes of this change in resistance have been discovered only during the past 25 years. Wesley H. Bateman took it a step further, making a connection between stress and resistance to absorption, or in more positive terms, a correspondence between serenity and an increased ability of the skin to absorb nutrients.

Gary, what is the science behind the *Tao of Music?*

We all know music can put us in a positive or negative frame of mind, even make us feel physically better or worse. Cellusonic music gives one the ability to control and reinforce positive thoughts and, in that sense, control the course of each day. Why not listen to music that aligns your body with frequencies found in nature, allowing you to exist in your healthiest and most youthful physical state? The creators of cellusonic music or the *Tao of Music* sought to answer just that question.

Researcher Wesley Bateman, sound engineer Allan Howarth, and I (as composer) came together to determine the frequencies that influence the tones, harmonics, and musical sequences providing the most benefit to human bodies and minds.

What we discovered is remarkable. Through the science of biofeedback and observing human brainwaves in relationship to the Schumann resonance (see page 119), we were able to compare and align musical tones with what ancient Buddhism calls "The Silent Sound of the Universe." Using the OM sound and the secrets of the "Music of the Spheres" referred to in the study of ancient pyramids, Bateman discovered the existence of a natural system of mathematics now called the "RA system."

During the course of Bateman's early studies, two well-known mathematical constants—π (pi) and U (phi)—were linked as never before to the brainwave frequencies produced by the four resonant systems of the human brain (delta, theta, alpha, and beta). In RA math, what are known as Fibonacci numbers, ratios, and logarithmic spirals are found in the shapes of plants, animals, and humans. One of them—pi or 3.14—is linked to higher levels of human perception. Another—phi or 1.618 or RA 1.62—is found throughout nature. By creating a keyboard coinciding with these mathematic and spiritual codes, we were able to make music harmonizing with these natural elements.

Cellusonic music resonates with your body through frequencies that occur in nature. Created entirely in tune with RA mathematics, it uses ELF waves and frequencies corresponding to higher levels of perception (see page 119), bringing you into sync with the natural frequencies of the earth and the objects around you.

The result is a 90-minute collection of music created with acoustic and electronic instruments (a sample is included with this volume). Each song is influenced by specific frequencies that calm the mind, enable accelerated healing in human cells, and improve one's overall sense of well-being.

Can the *Tao of Music* really make me calmer or help me to heal faster?

Just like heat and light, musical sound is a form of energy. Although no one can see music, its experiential properties are obvious. These range from an emotional response of feeling happy, sad, or invigorated, for instance, to a physical response such as tapping your toes or getting the shivers.

Any sound, including music, may be pleasant or unpleasant to the listener. We all have experienced excitement at hearing a dance beat, tension with eerie music, joy from uplifting music, and peace from calm music. There is no denying that music (sonic energy) affects us physically. In fact, music can profoundly affect both physical and mental health.

Users of the *Tao of Music* experience what they describe as "a slow awakening" or a sense of "infinite time"—like an opening of the mind in a space that is timeless. You don't have to make time for this music. It makes time for you.

How is the *Tao of Music* different from other music, especially New Age music that also claims to put listeners in an alpha state?

Two things distinguish it. First, you just do not get tired of this music. You can play it again and again. No matter how beautiful other music may be, you do tire of it. The *Tao of Music* passes through you, resonating with your cellular structure. Your brain recognizes its alpha waves and resonates on the same frequency.

Second, this music uses frequencies of a different standard timing calculated through a long research and discovery process. Its vibrations somehow awaken the pituitary and pineal glands (governing your cognitive, intellectual, and intuitive functions). It seems to awaken the average listener's inner self and soul. It seems to awaken autistic children from their cocoons.

Again, the *Tao of Music* aligns the mind with these natural frequencies to:

- relieve your stress and anxiety
- optimize your concentration, focus, and ability to learn
- improve your memory
- expand your creativity
- increase your motivation and boost your confidence
- provide a sense of "infinite time" and gradual spiritual awakening

- promote better chi in your internal organs
- contribute to your overall mental, spiritual, and physical health.

How did Wesley Bateman discover this special-frequency music?

While he was researching the topic of biofeedback training, a system that teaches a person to create alpha waves at will to control a particular physiological function (blood pressure, heart rate, muscle tension, or mental attitude, for instance), Wes came across a study called *The Schumann Resonances of the Earth-Ionosphere Cavity—Extremely Low Frequency Reception at Kingston Rhode Island.* This report documents the instrumentation used for retrieving and recording ELF, or extremely low-frequency waves. ELF wave trains produced by lightning strokes resonate in a natural cavity (wave-guide) composed of the earth's surface and ionosphere.

The frequencies and shapes of ELF waves and human waves are so alike that distinguishing between them is difficult. In fact, they have the same frequencies. When a person engages in meditation, he or she generates more alpha than other types of brainwaves. Since ELF waves with the frequencies of alpha brainwaves occur more often than others, it's logical to assume that naturally occurring ELF waves induce a state of tranquil meditation and eliminate stress. In other words, through listening to music with ELF waves, you gain the benefits of meditation without meditating! This music helps you tap into your universal life field.

What is a universal life field?

All forms of life live and have their being within the confines of an omnipresent, all-permeating Universal Lfe Field, or ULF. You become ill when your physical relationship to the ULF weakens. The body dies when it cannot maintain even the slightest physical relationship to the ULF. This relationship is evident in the biorhythms that all humans experience in cycles—a 23-day physical cycle, a 28-day emotional cycle, and a 33-day intellectual cycle—all having positive and negative phases.

Your ULF also includes four levels of perception—molar, micro, macro, and mega: all life as we know it lives within the three-dimensional molar (earth) level of perception. At this level, we use our five senses—hearing, tasting, seeing, smelling, and touching. The body and brain are molar-level objects, but the mind and spirit are not. The mind of a living person is based in the next level of perception—the micro level—of the ULF. The molar brain acts as a medium for the micro mind, providing the mind with the means to focus and express itself in the molar (earth) level.

Tao of Music resonates you into the higher, macro and mega, levels of the ULF.

What is resonance?

Resonance is the reinforcement of the natural vibration of a system or object by a force acting with the same frequency as the system. Every object or system has a natural frequency at which it will vibrate if it is displaced or distorted and released. In other words, frequencies of a feather flock together. When you hit middle C on the piano, for instance, the other C strings resonate with it even when you don't strike them. This principle applies to all vibrating bodies that send out energy waves—the human brain is one. Thus, human brainwaves similar to the ELF waves are stimulated by the continuous, naturally occurring ELF waves.

Upon discovering this, Wes's team set about testing subjects by synching their brainwaves with ELF waves. What we found is that subjects whose brainwaves were synched with ELF waves went into a deep, meditative, alpha state. After experiencing the calm and focus of an ELF-wave-induced alpha state for certain period, they felt a "burst" of energy from what they described as an unknown source.

These bursts showed up on the equipment measuring brainwave activity. In addition, a measurable, physical change occurred in the electrical conduction of the subject's skin. Imagine what these waves, in the form of music, could do for you!

Gary, how did you produce this music?

Though I have composed both *Artovan Music* and *Silent Visitation*, I have no background in music. It has something to do with my work in interior design. For more than 20 years I've been designing homes to harmonize with my clients' personalities. My method goes beyond design fads or even feng shui. I try to design interiors that synchronize with each homeowner's essence, through sensing the clients' energy and predicting what will best suit them. This translates well into making music.

Here's how: Most music is made of frequencies that bounce off the body, creating dissonance between the body and its surroundings. I sat down to a keyboard influenced by frequencies resonating with my body and just felt my way around the keys, sensing the energy within them and within my own body. The result is music made of frequencies that resonate with the human body. There is no disharmony.

How can I use this music?

Listening to cellusonic music can help you to feel relaxed and focused and elevate your mood, to achieve peace at the cellular level.

- Choose a time in the morning or evening to listen to this music, whichever time you're most likely to continue listening on a regular basis.
- Play the music CD in a standard CD player at your desired volume. in relaxed environment.
- Relax, clear your mind, and allow the music to wash through you.

After listening to this music for 10 minutes (the minimum recommended), you will feel relaxed, focused, and renewed, but listen for as long as you wish. Some prefer to play it in the background at the home or office all day, to soothe the subconscious mind and allow continued focus. Used in classrooms, it stimulates the mind and opens children with autism to interaction with the world around them.

The Power of the Music

Being in synch with the frequencies of nature brings you to an alpha state, a state of contentment. This natural contentment precludes seeking fulfillment from things that may harm the natural world or yourself. As I have said, I sit in my backyard and meditate, listening to the *Tao of Music*. In front of me are 16 small rocks placed to

A Critical Piece

Annie, our 11-year-old daughter, has mild autism. Her challenges are primarily in the areas of impulse control and interpersonal communication—not catching the subtleties of social interaction, not able to carry on extended conversation, and a tendency to repeat herself.

When we could not find answers in typical American medicine, we began to look outside the box. Our best information came from other parents, friends, and the Internet. At age 3, Annie started with alternative therapies such as infrared sauna sessions, energy balancing, the NAET method of allergy elimination, and a particular vitamin regimen.

We became aware of the positive effects that music therapy could have on children with auditory-processing issues and made good use of "A Chance To Grow" in Minneapolis and a program in Phoenix using "Tomatis" sound therapy. So, when a friend invited us to a home designed to enhance the effects of a particular set of sound frequencies, we were intrigued.

I had no idea what to expect. Annie and I arrived at a beautiful house with rounded room, high ceilings, and museum-like furnishings. I was nervous about her tendency to flit about, touching and feeling everything. The music, compiled on a CD, played softly as we entered. In the foyer, Annie stopped, looked around, and asked, "Is this a hotel?" We all laughed. Instead of tearing off, she walked slowly through the rooms. I was ready to stop her inevitable key-pounding when she approached the grand piano, but she walked around it, examining it carefully.

In the large oval room with a huge crescent-shaped couch and rounded coffee table, the effect of the music was dramatic. Annie sat next to me, quietly looking around. Next she climbed into my lap—a rarity at the time. She held up her hands, examining them, relaxed, calm. We sat there for almost an hour.

Since then Annie has listened to the full CD as she falls to sleep each night. Her impulsivity has decreased; focus and self-care have improved. Now she dresses herself, makes her own food, ask for help. The *Tao of Music* is a critical piece of our efforts to move Annie toward independence, self-awareness. and age-appropriate interaction.

—Kate Heegaard Hartfiel, Minneapolis

form an elliptical orb. I walk on the path of the orb. You might choose to meditate in this way or to find a path in the woods or in an urban park. While you walk, allow silence to teach you the lesson of contentment. Stop and close your eyes. Sink into the present moment through awareness of your body and your breathing. Turn attention to the sound of nature. Feel your connection to the landscape and its living being. I notice the squirrels and wild ducks and enjoy a sense of oneness with creation.

Everything in the universe transmits an energy through the universe. Every person, animal, plant, rock, tree—every physical being—sends out energy like a radio transmitter. The Chinese people call this energy, especially the energy flowing between cells, "chi." You are sending out energy now, from the center of your being, in all directions. You are this energy, and you move outward in wave patterns. The energy leaves you, moves through walls, over buildings, past the continent, and into the forever, and it never stops. Have you ever felt the need to contact a person out of the blue? Have you entered a room where you feel negative energy or a joyful room where people are laughing? These feelings are the result of chi.

The energy you feel depends on the energy of the people and the shape of the room and its decoration. When I walk into the Grand Hyatt Hotel in Hong Kong, I feel a new sense of energy. I am drawn to look at the ceiling—the entrance is a huge elliptical orb, like the pattern of the stones in my backyard. A feng-shui master must have suggested that shape to bring a certain energy to the hotel. You can feel it the minute you walk in.

The same is true of the entrance to the observatory at Rockefeller Center in New York. When you stand inside the entrance looking up, you feel a vibration with the crystals hanging from the orb-shaped ceiling there.

Every thought in your mind has energy. Every word you say shapes it. Every deed you do affects it. The vibration, speed, wavelength, and frequency of your chi changes constantly with your thoughts, moods, feelings, words, and actions. Be sure you sending out positive, joyful, compassionate, and contented chi.

All the world exchanges energy all the time. Your energy pushes out, touching everything else. Everything and everyone touches you. The air between you and your

Connection

My son John was born cocaine-dependent to a drunk mother and suffered a brain bleed in the first day of his life. He lived in a foster home, locked in a room for the first 3½ years of his life. He processes things very slowly—change and learning are at a snail's pace. He is, or I should say we are, in a treatment program because he has reactive attachment disorder. He exhibits oppositional, defiant behaviors and is fairly self-defeating.

Several months ago, John started listening to your music. We play it when he is falling asleep. If he is particularly difficult, I turn it on again in the morning . . . so he can wake up to it. The first time he listened [there was] a dramatic change in his behavior. He was able to talk with me for a long period of time about his difficulty in living with us and about the things he does to push us away.

When we started our summer routine I forgot about the music . . . John began to attend a summer day camp, which is a part of the treatment program. The camp activities address his behaviors and are designed to encourage attachment. The challenges to make changes were demanding, and he reverted to his old behaviors . . .

A few weeks ago, I started playing the music again. Just as before, he is beginning to think more clearly and to process information. Without the music, he seems unable to make connections between his behavior and other people's reactions to him . . . I am thankful for this music.

—Mary

environment fills with this energy. The intertwining chi forms the collective chi or consciousness we call "the matrix." The weave of combined energy is powerful, and it affects everything. The ancients understood that, and they discovered that the sound OM could be used to change the energy and achieve an alpha state in the brain. The Tibetan monks chant OM to attain such a state—nirvana.

By taking time to meditate, to be with nature through this music, you contribute to a positive, powerful, dynamic matrix, immersing yourself in the natural beauty of the land, renewing your loving relationship with the earth, and sharing your contentment with the world.

Galvanic Skin Response

Stressed skin contracts and thus resists therapy. A person's general mood as well as his or her immediate reaction to a stimulus determines the degree of resistance. A simple psycho-galvanometer was the earliest tool used to measure the resistance of the skin to the passage of a current. Tarchanoff wrote on this subject in 1890, but only within the last 25 years have the underlying causes of changes in resistance been discovered.

You have all heard of lie detectors, which measure physical response (galvanic skin response) as a clue to whether or not a person is telling the truth. The concept has also been used to measure emotional response during therapy sessions.

The Tarchanoff, or galvanic skin, response is related to the level of arousal of the cortex of the brain. The emotional charge of hearing a specific word may affect that level, causing a response. Because the human hand has so many nerve endings on the sensorimotor strip of the cortex of the brain, handheld electrodes are ideal for indicating response. As arousal increases, the fight-or-flight response of the autonomic nervous system occurs. Adrenaline causes increased sweating, for example. Sweating, however, is nowhere near so instantaneous or accurate as the galvanic skin response. The most advanced layers of the cortex, unique to humans, link to the thumb and forefinger especially, resulting in a further, complex physiological response to arousal of the forebrain. Changes in alpha rhythms cause blood capillaries to enlarge, also affecting response.

By virtue of the galvanic skin response, autonomic nervous system activity causes a change in the skin's conductivity. A rise or fall relates directly to reactive arousal, due to restimulation of repressed mental conflict. Initially this may cause a rise in resistance. When the conflict is resolved through the viewing of objective reality—the truth of exact time, place, form, and event—the emotional charge dissipates, and the release of energy reduces resistance.

Powerful Stuff!

Tao of Music is different from other New Age music—it really puts you into a relaxed, alpha-brainwave state. You just do not get tired of this music. We have played this before and after each class for more than a year. The music awakens the inner self and the soul of the average listener. The plants are thriving, and all the yogis who come to our studio seem happier and stay longer when we play the music there.

—Laiki Huxorli and Herb Kearse
Owners and Instructors
Bikram's Yoga College of India
Bloomington, MN

The Swiss psychologist Carl Jung, in perhaps the earliest practical use of the theory, connected subjects to an instrument measuring changes in the resistance of the skin. He read to them specific words, one by one, to determine which lines of enquiry were most likely to be fruitful for each subject. But without amplification, his device remained little more than a laboratory curiosity. Once a portable psycho-galvanometer with amplification became available, criminologists picked up the idea with enthusiasm, and police forces have used lie detectors for the past 60 years. Little further work with psycho-galvanometers occurred until biofeedback research on meditation and relaxation employed it in the 1970s.

Biofeedback makes possible an individual's self-regulation of awareness states. Cortical arousal level is central to a person's level of awareness, and a machine measuring this factor was critical. The most important findings of the research of the past 25 years are:

1. A low level of cortical arousal is desirable for relaxation, hypnosis, and the subjective experience of psychic states and unconscious manifestations.
2. A high level of cortical arousal gives increased powers of reflection, focused concentration, reading speed, and capacity for long-term recall.
3. Cortical arousal has a simple relationship to skin conductivity. Arousal of the cortex increases the conductivity of the skin, and a drop in arousal causes a drop in skin conductivity. With a few hours' practice with a sensitive meter, a person can consciously control the level of arousal over wide limits.

Volney Mathison was a pioneer in the discovery that all fears, feelings, resentments, all thought and emotion, are electrical in nature. He found in his 1940s lie-detector experiments that when a person was reminded of certain past events or induced with a change of mood, the needle in the meter jumped in proportion to the strength of unconscious reaction. In skilled hands, the meter could be used to locate particular mental content, its nature, location in space and time, and amount of force. Mathison's research made it possible for him to invent the portable transistorized GSR meter and to develop a list of words triggering responses associated with fear or resentment.

Biofeedback research shows that meditation and relaxation cause a rise in skin resistance and has assumed that high skin resistance indicates a pleasant, relaxed state of mind and low resistance indicates tension. But the reverse is true in psychotherapy. When repressed material—associated with guilt or fear, for example—comes to the surface, skin resistance rises, and when the guilt or fear discharges, it drops in relief.

Michael J. Apter of Bristol University referred to this phenomenon in his book *Reversal Theory* as "paradoxical arousal." He wrote that high arousal is pleasant and exciting when a person is in the active state but unpleasant when he or she is in the thinking state. A person with a traumatic history experiences high arousal as unpleasant: cortical arousal is unequal due to restimulation (evident on a bilateral GSR meter). But when cortical arousal is uniform, a person experiences a pleasant state of high energy.

This is similar to Sigmund Freud's early finding that high arousal in a neurotic person is experienced as unpleasant internal excitement, whereas a person substantially free from neurosis experiences arousal as energy for incitement, or action. Our own findings substantiate Freud's—with erasure or transcendence of fear and guilt comes greater capacity to operate at high arousal, in a relaxed state, and at a high emotional tone.

To resolve the paradox, we suggest correlating high and low skin resistance, not with relaxation and stress but with withdrawal and involvement, respectively. Both of the latter terms may refer to both relaxed and tense states. The state of withdrawal is relaxed when it means detachment from worldly cares or abandoning responsibility; it is tense when it means an inability to confront repressed material. Involvement is tense when it means overreach or anxiety and relaxed when it means enhanced awareness or when there is a flash of insight and the sudden clearing of mental blockage caused by guilt or fear.

Biofeedback researcher Wesley Bateman has said, "It is widely known in the scientific community that certain emotional stress will change the physiological state of the skin . . . this electrical resistance in the skin can limit or counteract the therapeutic effectiveness of lotions or biological formulations that could assist in the healing process."

The bottom line is that cellusonic music induces relaxation, and relaxation decreases the resistance of the skin to treatment. So my sister Cathy and I, after applying our Biolaxin™ (relaxin) cream each night, listen to this music to achieve optimum absorption. At the very least, in giving yourself this quiet time, you allow yourself to listen to your soul and relax into a good night's sleep.

The Phoenix—Living Feng Shui

The phrase *feng shui* means wind and water. Many of you are aware of the use of feng shui in interior design. In that popular translation of its use, however, feng shui loses its essence. Aside from both that and the textbook explanation, I grew up living the idea of feng shui: I learned the concept from my father and the villagers in Taipo Market—a place with good feng shui, a spot of the best convergence of good chi.

The world's natural convergence of landscape provides feng shui as well. If you pay attention, you can know good feng shui from the exchange of your vibrations with the world around you. Certain shapes provide that vibration. You become a feng shui master as you become attuned with the chi around you. Certain kinds of food (gluten and casein) fill you with toxins, and you lose this chi. But if you eat properly, your internal chi flows, sending out better vibrations. You become an intuitive eater, finding food that sings to you and that your body sings about after you eat it. Develop this sensibility, and you will learn to respond to your landscape in a similar way.

As a child, I watched the Man family–a clan of more than 30—posed for a portrait in front of our house in Taipo Market. The head of the clan hardly ever stepped outside his home, yet he came all the way to our house for that photo, wearing the formal mandarin outfit saved for special occasions. I asked my father why they picked the spot in front of our house. He said that the old man agreed to come only because that spot had good feng shui.

Later I learned that the members of the Man family are descendents of the last prime minister of the Sung Dynasty, who died in prison because he would not yield to the Mongols. His descendents left for the Tai Po area and settled there for more than 500 years. They had lived as farmers, close to the land; they knew about feng shui. (Be sure, when you visit Hong Kong, to see the Man family's ancestral memorial in Tai Po. Prime Minister Man's most famous poem is carved on the wall there.)

My father told me that he had learned about feng shui from Ah Ma and the villagers. Once he said to me, " May, you are a phoenix that plays a flute!" I answered, "What do you mean by that?" and he told me a story I will never forget:

Ah Ma was looking for a burial plot for herself and her children. (The Chinese believe that the place where they are buried affects their descendents.) Ah Ma took a risk in creating a new life for herself and her son and grandchildren, and she wanted to be sure that the generations to come would do as well. She found a spot for burial and asked a feng shui master to check it out. He said the land was good. When she was buried there, she would face the brook that ran by the burial plot. The brook made a beautiful sound, like a phoenix playing a flute.

"Your female line will prosper if you are buried in this spot," he said. "Are you sure this is the spot?" She answered: "This is just fine. I would like my female line to play the flute and make beautiful music."

My father said, "See, May, you are the phoenix that plays the flute." So when I sit or walk to the *Tao of Music* in my backyard, I feel the exchange of vibrations—the orb, my trees, my lake, the good chi of those and of my Ah Ma. I am the phoenix playing beautiful music. I have not left my Ah Ma's lap.

The Holy Grail and the *Tao of Youth*

Why do I put those two topics together? You should know by now that I like to tell stories and to put unlikely ideas together. Three years ago I went back to Hong Kong to work with high-school classmates to plan a 40-year class reunion. I traveled to Hong Kong by myself, on the way reading *The Da Vinci Code*. I stayed at a friend's apartment and spent every free moment reading that book.

Intrigued with the concept of the Holy Grail in that book, I began to look for other writings on the subject. What were the stories behind the myth? And why has the myth continued for so many years? Soon I came across *The Holy Grail: It Origins, Secrets and Meaning Revealed* by Malcolm Godwin. He summarized some of the origins of these myths, which he had traced from Celtic to Christian legends.

What is the grail? And what is it supposed to do? Most of the tales and legends center on two concepts—the grail as a dish, chalice, or cup used at the Last Supper of Christian origin or the grail as Mary Magdalene's tomb, or Jesus' blood. The quest has been as varied as the vessel sought—a search for the ultimate source, for rebirth, for the fountain of youth, the settling of feuds, or the renewal of self. The quest and the grail are intertwined.

After reading Malcolm's summaries of the tales, I realized that I have been on a quest myself—a journey to find out about myself and to find the truth. As I read the stories, I noticed a common thread—each tells of a knight who has raised himself, who is socially awkward, the odd man out, but actively engaged in a quest. Sometimes he is seen as a fool because he asks so many unusual questions and approaches a situation or turn of events with pure focus.

My brother Sam is one of those knights, like Perceval (piercing the valley), who keeps asking questions and goes about his quest single-mindedly, not merely or passively listening to and accepting the ideas of others but marching to the beat of his own drum. In the legends, this type—not the other knights—ends up finding the grail. That is how Sam found relaxin—what we have also called the Cinderella hormone or the fountain of youth. In this context, I'd call Sam the Eastern knight (even though we earlier compared him to a fairy godmother!).

Now in Key 4 to the *Tao of Youth*, I introduce to you another—Gary, the Western knight. Gary, like Sam and Perceval, has found a tool that helps meet a need, in this case one that provides for a peaceful and spiritual state of mind. In all three cases, the quest has transformed the knight, who also has discovered himself, become enlightened, and in doing so has become a hero. The stories of the quests that brought Sam and Gary to the vessels are in themselves worthy of separate books.

I understand that you might say, "May, you are kind of crazy bringing these unrelated concepts together," even more so when I suggest that the Eastern culture's pursuit of Quan Yin parallels the pursuit of the Virgin Mary in the West. Whether from East or West, we all yearn for inner peace and paradise. We always have, from ancient times to the present. We all ask, "Why do we exist? What can we do in this world to find peace within ourselves? What is the truth?" That's what I am doing; I am in search of those answers, my grail, and I write this book as part of my journey.

In Malcolm Godwin's book is a tale about Perceval and another knight who discovered that the Holy Grail was not the cup from which Jesus drank wine at the Last Supper but the food that Jesus served to the disciples there. That was the innermost secret—the Holy Grail.

Michelangelo's painting of the Last Supper as shown in the movie *The Da Vinci Code* shows no cup but only an elliptically shaped platter (as knight Gary has pointed out to me).

After reading that passage of Godwin's book, I wondered whether the fountain of youth mentioned in tales and myths was about the food offered and not about the blood of Jesus Christ. The food we eat turns into the blood that nourishes our bodies that gives us that joyful feeling that Parzival (Perceval) discovered in the legend by Wolfram Von Eschenbach more than a century ago.

In that story, the food on the platter and the drink in the cup are the ultimate transformation of the knight and his country. Every story is about the quest to restore the wasteland to paradise, and that is what we are trying to do here. The best food and drink for your body and soul will restore you to paradise—that is the *Tao of Youth*.

Key 5

Understanding your largest organ: Skincare from the inside out

What's Inside?

Most people don't think of their skin as their largest organ—or as an organ at all. Yet skin is both a protector (you can't do without it) and an indicator of health, not to mention an indicator of your age. Most women are willing to spend thousands of dollars and many hours taking care of their external skin, paying little attention to their inner organs.

But skin is so important, once you think about it, that you may wonder why we've left it to the end. The truth is, if you practice the things we've discussed so far, your skin is already beautiful. Understanding a bit more about taking care of it from the inside out will make it as good as it can be.

When people talk about skin, they're usually referring only to the outside skin. But skin, the largest organ in your body, lines your insides as well, protecting your internal organs from a toxic world. How does your inner skin affect your outside skin?

Keys 1 and 5 are interrelated. You might think of it as coming full circle. We have emphasized the importance of the digestive system. We have introduced food that nourishes the digestive system rather than overloading it. You are what you digest.

When we say "inner skin" we mean the wall of the gastrointestinal tract, which begins at the mouth, travels through the stomach, intestines, colon, and ends at the rectum. Many people are willing to spend hundreds of dollars at a spa for facial treatments but ignore and abuse their digestive systems constantly. Abuse of the inner skin affects the inner body, and its diminished function results in the rapid aging of the outside skin. To achieve a healthy glow on the outside, you must pay as much attention to the digestive system.

Why talk about digestion when Key 5 is about skin? I noticed that after I faithfully implemented the food strategies meant to lose water weight that my skin glowed. In fact, other people asked me about it. A harmonious digestive system means the proper absorption of nutrients, and it shows on your face. Dr. Sam Yue explains:

Why do we eat? To gather building blocks for the body and to supply it with energy. Digestion is the process that breaks the food into molecules so that the nutrients can reach every cell. Larger particles become smaller, become absorbable and usable as they reduce in size. Carbohydrates become glucose. Proteins become polypeptides become amino acids. Lipids become fatty acids. Nucleic acids become nucleotides.

The digestive system starts all this work in the mouth. Your chewing breaks down the food mechanically (with your jaws and teeth). Saliva breaks starch into glucose with the enzyme amylase. Then the food travels (through smooth-muscle contraction in the throat and esophagus) to your stomach. The acids in the stomach help pepsin break proteins into peptides. Enzymes secreted from the walls of the duodenum and pancreas, plus bile from the gall bladder and liver, break it down further.

Finally, in the small intestine, which is eight meters long and contains the same enzymes, most of the food is digested and absorbed through millions of villi (little fingers). The large intestine absorbs water and electrolytes (sodium is one). The microbes there break and ferment anything that's left, and the rectum stores any solid waste until it is excreted through the anus.

The touchiest parts of the system are the stomach and the small and large intestines. The small intestine is the site of the Leaky Gut Syndrome discussed in Key 1. Every part of the system, including the inner skin, must be healthy for it to work properly. Everything you can do to take care of it will serve you well.

The Enzymes Story

Taking care of your digestive system is essential to your health and to your skin. For the long run that means enzyme supplementation. I've attended antiaging conferences for a number of years, often conversing with physicians who have successfully used enzymes to treat various patient complaints. European medicine is far more advanced than American medicine in understanding how powerful enzymes can be.

I read Marilyn Diamond and Donald B. Schnell's book *Fitonics® for Life* about ten years ago. What they wrote still makes sense to me. Diamond sums it up—enzymes are the life action in every living thing. The word "enzymes" means "to ferment" or "to cause a change." Enzymes are (protein) catalysts for the body's biochemical processes. You cannot run, walk, breathe, or blink without enzymes. You cannot see, hear, think, move a muscle, or have sex without them. You cannot digest your food, repair your cells, or cleanse your body without them, either. Without enzymes, life could not exist. They are the tools that create life. All living material contains enzymes; they control the chemical reactions of all organisms. More than 3,000 enzymes have been discovered in the human body. There are 98 enzymes enabling specific tasks in the arteries alone.

Your body does not have an unlimited supply of enzymes. In fact, you inherit your ability to manufacture enzymes at birth; the capacity for producing them is unique to each individual. Whatever that capacity, it diminishes with age.

Conserving enzymes is a key to health and weight loss. Eating foods that contain large amounts of enzymes—(for example, raw fruits and vegetables)—maintains your enzyme "savings account." If you supply the enzymes you need from other sources, you don't have to use up all you have or can produce yourself. The digestion of food requires more enzymes than any other single body process. Relieving this burden—by supplementing the enzymes needed for digestion—allows the body to produce enzymes for other necessary functions such as fighting viruses and repairing cells.

Supplementing digestive enzymes is important because we cook much of our food at temperatures higher than 118 degrees F.—at which point many enzymes die. That's why eating a lot of raw fruits and vegetables works. That's why we recommend juicing and Oolong tea in the morning. Both fruit and tea contain many enzymes and antioxidants.

Wobenzym®, a combination of animal and vegetable enzymes and the biggest over-the counter-food supplement in Germany, is commonly used in "systemic enzymes treatment." My brother Sam recommends taking Wobenzym® during meals, to ease digestion. I have been doing this for a number of years. (See *The Aspirin Alternative* (systemic oral enzymes) by Michael Loes, and Dr. Sam's enzyme supplement list, on page 138–39.)

The Glyconutrient Story

Health at the cellular level is particularly important to skin and as part of the health capital plan described in Key 1. Recent scientific discoveries have revealed a new class of nutrients necessary for life: glyconutrients for cell-to-cell communication. These are specific sugars (found in nature) essential to the function and structure of the human body.

We would like to get the glyconutrients we need from what we eat—from fresh, ripe fruits and vegetables. But because of general farming and food-prepartion practices, at least six of the eight glyconutrients are not available in our diets today (see MIT's "Reclaiming Your Health Starts at the Cell Level with Glyconutrients," in the February 2003 issue of *Technology Review*).

In addition to improving cell-to cell communication, research shows, these sugars are the monosaccharides, or simple sugars, that regulate, defend, protect, and repair cells. (Four of the last eight Nobel Prizes in Physiology have gone to researchers working on cellular communication and how these sugars work in the body).

Eight Necessary Glyconutrients (Sugars)

1. mannose
2. fucose
3. galactose
4. glucose
5. N-acetylgalactosamine
6. N-acetylglucosamine
7. N-acetylneuraminic acid
8. xylose

A basic understanding of the immune system is useful. The major components of the immune system are the:

- thymus gland, which produces the T cells that are part of white blood cells
- spleen, which filters foreign cells from the blood
- lymph system, a complex system helping to bathe blood plasma with nutrients and to filter out bacteria and viruses
- antibodies, which bind to toxins to stop their movement through the body
- hormones, which encourage white-blood-cell production.

Each of these systems of cell groups must be strong to help to kill enemy or mutant cells, stop infection, and heal wounds. And, if the communication between cells breaks down, the immune system cells may not know, for example, about a virus invading the lungs or liver, a fungus taking over the digestive tract, or that a cluster of cancer cells is rapidly reproducing in a breast. These eight simple sugars act as the major operating system so that all the other systems can work together.

Enzymes: Essence of Life

Your health depends on a balance of metabolic and digestive enzymes. The ability to produce digestive enzymes decreases with age. By age 50 you lose about 40 percent of that capacity. Food devoid of enzymes or otherwise hard to digest diverts the body's resources to produce digestive enzymes at the expense of metabolic enzymes. As a result, other body functions suffer, and well-being flies out the window.

To counter the aging process:
* Eat as much raw, colorful fruit and vegetables as possible for their plant enzymes, bioflavonoids, and antioxidants, which assist digestion. Canning, cooking, and processing destroy these beneficial enzymes and nutrients.
* Avoid hard-to-digest ingredients like gluten and casein.
* Use juicing and tea as natural ways to increase enzymes and thus reduce lymphedema.
* Supplement with plant and animal enzymes to help digestion and reduce conditions predisposing you to chronic disease.

For digestion (for general purposes, choose an enteric-coated product, preventing action until it reaches the intestines; choose non-enteric-coated products for action in the stomach):

Plant-based enzymes (many derived from fungi) include:
* papain (found in papaya)
* rutin (found in buckwheat)
* bromelain (found in pineapple)

Animal-based enzymes include:
* amylase (to digest carbohydrate)
* protease (to digest protein)
* lipase (to digest fat)

(continued opposite)

Over-the-counter enzymes:
- Wobenzym® (one of the best enteric-coated, general-purpose enzymes)

Prescription (enteric-coated) enzymes:
- Creon®
- Ultrase® MT20
- Generic MT20 (pancrelipase)

Beyond Digestion
To reduce lymphedema and increase immunity:
- Wobenzym® N (5–8 tablets on an empty stomach twice daily)

To reduce lymphedema, increase immunity, and break down mucus in the lung linings (check with your physician first if you are taking Coumadin®):
- seaprose (30 mg twice daily)
- serratiopeptidase (34 mg or 20,000 units once in the morning)

Herbs to reduce lymphedema and break down mucus:
- horse-chestnut seed (extract aecin, 60 mg twice daily)
- hesperidin (flavonoid, 50 mg twice daily)
- diosmin (flavonoid, 450 mg twice daily, usually combined with hesperidin) guaifenesin (600 mg twice daily for sustained release; or 400 mg three or four times daily)

This concept is the overarching, heretofore missing, link in our quest for health capital enough to maintain healthy bodies for as long as we can. If you eat well, such as with the *Tao of Youth* plan, and supplement judiciously with vitamins and minerals, chances are you have most of the bases covered. This result of the newest research, however, suggests that supplementing the eight glyconutrients is a good idea too. There are other products, but I personally supplement with a small scoop of Ambrotose™ from Mannatech, Inc., in my morning juice. My rationale for supplementing? I have not raised any of the fruits or vegetables, and they are likely to have been picked too early to develop all the glyconutrients I need.

How I Got to This Point

By now you know that I am curious about every aspect of my life. My role models—mostly family—encouraged me to question things, even when I was a child.

I didn't pay much attention to appearance then—I was the first girl after three boys. In Taipo Market, at that time a quiet town outside Kowloon, we coexisted with the fishermen who lived in boats about a five-minute walk from our home and with the local farming people who settled there more than 500 years ago, when the Mongolians drove out the last emperor of the Sung Dynasty. (The guards and the child emperor jumped into the ocean, taking their lives. You can visit the rock from which they jumped into the sea). The descendents of the guards and the famous General Man (including one of my best friends) lived not far from our house.

Outside Kowloon and far from Hong Kong, Taipo Market had few Western healthcare facilities when we lived there in the 1950s and 1960s. My father was the only Western-trained physician in the eastern region of the New Territories, which included a vast area of the Hong Kong territory adjacent to China. We were outsiders in this area much like rural mainland China after it closed its borders.

Since Hong Kong was a colony of Great Britain, my father often interacted with the British government in his work. My brothers and sister and I grew up there with a lot of freedom and fun, absorbing cultural differences. We were the last generation to have a taste of what it was like to grow up there under British rule and at the same time experience such a diverse mix of people.

What does this has to do with skincare? I feel my upbringing set the tone for my curiosity. Even my later schoolmates in Hong Kong grew up with a different experience—they lived in concrete buildings while I ran in fields of watercress and played with jellyfish in the boats of the fishermen, who were also my father's patients.

There were disadvantages in our remoteness. We did not have dental care until I was 12 years old. I still blame my father, who substituted as our dentist, for pulling out only part of my baby teeth—one tooth grew in crooked, and I lost two others to decay. But outside of that, I would not trade my childhood for any other.

I was more interested in following my three older brothers in their explorations than in staying at home to sew or play with dolls. We trapped crabs and fished in the mountain streams. Every day there was something new. The boys loved climbing on the high piles of tree branches that local farmers gathered for cooking fuel. As the youngest, I had the toughest time climbing to the platform where they played at sword fighting, as they had seen in Western movies playing at the local theater. The women farmers (who did all the work while the men took their birds to the market and sat around) chased us out, smacking my brothers' heads when they did not run fast enough to get out of the way. As the smallest of my siblings, and a girl, I came out unscathed.

At about age 12, I finished grade school and first experienced the British educational system in Hong Kong. I matriculated at a lower school, then the upper school for high school. My mother was determined to change me into a feminine girl. She was tired of my tomboy activities. The last straw was my falling into the sea at age 10 (over an embankment of about 20 feet onto oyster rocks and muddy sand), while they were out of town.

I was lucky—my bicycle and I landed between two oyster-filled rocks. The whole town came to see the dead girl, but I was simply embarrassed at being covered with black mud, not hurt at all. My brothers had just handed me the bike and forgotten to show me how to use the brakes. I had always just followed them on my tricycle.

Entering an all-girl school meant I was to learn everything about being a girl, to become the young woman my mother thought I should become. Fortunately for me, the school she sent me to was and still is one of the best schools in the colony. It was unusual in its focus on challenging the intellect and curious minds of its female students. Many alumnae of the Diocesan Girls' School, run by the Anglican Church, have gone on to become leaders in Hong Kong or other parts of the world.

So my experiences in childhood and at school provided the background that has led me to question my life and whatever I am doing. The sophistication of the cosmetic counters and jewelry and clothing stores in every other street of Hong Kong brought me to a new consciousness of how I appeared to others. I learned about quality and variety and was influenced by European and other cultures. I began to like dressing like a girl and learning about how to be attractive.

I inherited good skin—from my aunt I've been told—so for many years I went along giving it little attention, wearing little makeup. All I did was wash my face with soap and water and apply a little lotion, and my skin was clear and soft and luminous. But at age 29 I began to see dryness and the first sign of wrinkles on my face. What could I do?

The answer was my usual one—use my inquisitive mind. Try to find out how well-known beauties have kept their skin beautiful. I read many books about skincare, then came across one about Erno Laszlo, whose skincare regime has been used by beauties such as Jacqueline Kennedy Onassis, Katherine Hepburn, Audrey Hepburn, and others. By the time I hit 30, I had decided to use his line of skincare products, and I adhered to that regimen for years.

Erno Laszlo

I have used Erno Laszlo's skincare regimen since I was 30 years old. I noticed my skin becoming dry and flaky in my late twenties and started searching for the best skincare program. What Dr. Erno Laszlo advocated in his approach to skincare made a lot of sense to me. I noticed his roster of clients—many well-known beauties—and started clipping photos of these women at that time. I thought, "If these women I admire all use his products, I will too." And so I have done that for many years.

Erno Laszlo is a legend, a pioneer in developing customized skin products for women in as early as the 1930s. According to Diana Lewis Jewell in *Angel of Beauty: The Story of Dr. Erno Laszlo*, he wrote: "The human skin leads a life of its own. It breathes, thinks, and it works. But at the same time, it registers all that you feel: fear, joy, horror, pain, and astonishment. It blushes with shame, it pales with fury. So much is written about the skin. But underneath it all, there is the glow, the original beauty nature gave you."

He stressed that beauty was the sole purpose of satisfying oneself, first and foremost. It must be inner directed, not the opposite. Happiness is the "best beauty lotion." Further, he wrote, "Beauty is an exquisite, flamelike miracle, ignited from the inside, not the outside."

And, he wrote: "Flirting is a marvelous beauty treatment for a woman. It stimulates the mysterious gland that makes the essential harmony between a woman's outlook on life and her appearance. Flirting makes her heart beat faster, stimulating the blood stream and thereby clearing the skin of blemishes, brightening her eyes, and even adding a gloss to her hair. Modern science, studying the relationship between the glandular system and the emotions, recognizes that the thrills and excitement of new attachment . . . are actually beauty aids."

Laszlo advocated proper eating, not starvation diets and unorthodox exercise. He advocated water for washing dirt from your face. He introduced essential fatty acids and other formulations as treatments for skin. His ideas prompted me to follow his skincare regimen, and I still think his ideas make sense. I think I was ahead of the curve, that I chose wisely a course on which I enjoyed good skin for many years. To have good skin when you are older, you must start young, he said. Aging well is a lifelong practice.

An investment in aging well is as important as investing financially for your retirement. Without good health, you will not be able to enjoy life, no matter how much money you might have.

We now know more about the inner and outer skin that we did in Laszlo's day, but the principle remains the same. Adding music to the equation aids meditation and so helps the layers of the derma absorb the benefits of the cream you use. The skin cannot lie; you cannot be beautiful without taking care of your skin from the inside out, without integrating mind, body, and spirit—a prerequisite for true health.

What You Put on Your Face

I used Erno Laszlo's night cream for about 30 years before its effects diminished. Much research had been done on the ingredients in skincare products since I began using that line, so I started to read up on those that might help my aging skin. I don't pretend to know everything about skincare products—I'm not a chemist—but I try to keep up on what might be useful to me.

When I read Dr. Nicholas Perricone's books, I was impressed by his advice to eat healthy food and take food supplements as a means to healthy and beautiful skin. And I started checking into the ingredients of newer cosmetic creams. This list includes currently popular ingredients available in most cosmetic products today:

Antioxidants
- Vitamin C-ester is vitamin C with an attached fatty acid. It is fat-soluble and rapidly penetrates the skin. Products containing vitamin C-ester are helpful in reducing and preventing skin damage. Vitamin C inhibits skin-damaging free radicals. It helps collagen synthesis, which declines in aging because of diminishing microcapillary circulation. Vitamin C regenerates vitamin E in the skin and enables it to provide sustainable antioxidant protection. The studies of vitamins C and E convince me they are essential ingredients in topical skin products.
- Alpha-lipoic acid is an antioxidant important in managing Type 2 diabetes. It is found in microchondria, the powerhouses of the cell. Alpha-lipoic acid decreases glycation (attachment of glucose to proteins), decreases pore size, and activates AP1 for healing. The result is a decrease in facial lines.

- Alpha- and beta-hydroxy acid, available for about 20 years, achieves a marked improvement in skin quality through exfoliative action—the removal of dead skin cells. Topical application of these fruit acids reduce fine lines and wrinkles and lend fresh tone to the skin.
- DMAE stabilizes cell membranes and addresses the sag of tissues caused by the destruction of the skin's underlying support structure (collagen and elastin). The result is firmer skin.
- Vitamin A and its retinoid analogue stimulate cell renewal by increasing the rate of mitotic cell division. It acts as a signaling agent to stimulate the binding of epidermal growth factor to skin cells.

Moisture in Skin

Most commercial face creams are oil-based and work by blocking the release of water from the skin. As we age we lose the ability to attract moisture and become dehydrated. The skin must be replenished with its natural moisturizer complex to attract and retain water. The following ingredients, applied topically, offer optimal protection: NaPCA, hyaluronic acid, lactic acid, urea, CEraphyl GA-D, and squalene.

Vitamin D

We get vitamin D naturally from sunlight, but the sun can also cause damage, even cause skin cancer. So get most of your vitamin D orally, in high dosage—1,400 IU daily—to prevent other kinds of cancer.

Thyroid Function

As we age we produce less thyroid hormone, leaving the skin dry, flaky, and sluggish. Seaweed, seafood, and fish are good remedies. I supplement that with Iodoral®.

Hormones and Skin

The sleep hormone (melatonin) and the antistress hormone (DHEA), both found in human skin, convert to other entities. DHEA becomes estrogen and androgen-type metabolites found only in skin. Melatonin is synthesized in skin, and in low concentration it can stimulate cell growth. Women who take estrogen and testosterone have been found to have thicker skin than those who do not. DHEA converts to both estrogen and testosterone, providing the benefits of both hormones. DHEA has powerful skin-protection effects. Melatonin is an antioxidant hormone protecting against UV radiation.

Skin is affected by many entities inside and out. Eat well, sleep well, and reduce stress to be sure your skin radiates your good health.

While I was reading up on how to take care of my skin, my brother Sam, the curious doctor, was learning more about the Chinese herbs that help people with skin problems. He noticed that many of his patients had skin problems, some with severe psoriasis. He mixed some cream obtained from the compound pharmacist with relaxin (the Cinderella hormone) and two Chinese herbs, provided the cream to those patients, and took before-and-after photos. After he showed me those photographs, we began documenting the results and found that with application of the cream, the skin with psoriasis ended up looking better than the skin around it. Since I am a vain, aging woman, I said to my brother, "Why don't you put the relaxin together with the ingredients I found in my research? I will be your guinea pig."

We hadn't yet thought about how to be sure the ingredients would penetrate the skin. Relaxin is a molecule bigger than the pores. So how could we be sure the ingredients would be absorbed? After some looking, we found a technology called cyclomethicone skin penetration, which pushes the pores sideways so that bigger ingredients can slide in. Problem solved.

Still, the cream didn't feel right, and it was "smelly" from the Chinese herbs. I told Sam that he didn't have a clue as to how fussy women are about texture and fragrance. After several tries, he got it right. When I told him it was perfect, he smiled and said he had taken some of the wild camellia-seed oil (see page 149) that he had found on my desk and put it into the cream. That made the texture heavenly. Now our company manufactures this cream. My sister and my friends and I have used it regularly for a couple of years. We feel good and look good—our skin glows.

In researching the key ingredient relaxin, we found clinical studies of its use in treating scleroderma in the 1950s and others showing that relaxin helps people with peripheral vascular disease. Dr. Christian Schwabe, who studied the effects of porcine relaxin for 35 years, found that the first sign of aging was "hardening of the arteries" as it was called in those days.

You probably have noticed that many pregnant women seem to glow—that is because of the increased microcirculation in their blood vessels due to increased relaxin in their systems during pregnancy. Freer blood flow provides the glow. Relaxin also causes thickening of the epidermis by stimulating cell division and renewal at a rate typical of younger skin, leading to the prevention of fine wrinkles.

I still use Erno Laszlo's skin cleansing regimen, though now I use wild camellia-seed oil before washing with the cleanser. Afterwards, my skin feels clean and moisturized. I also discovered an eye serum in China that I used regularly—the essence of the saffron flower grown in the high altitudes of Tibet. This combination works!

While I recommend your doing the same, I'll nag a bit like my mother and remind you that only 20 percent of a good skin result can be attributed to the application of any topical cream. If your skin is beautiful, most of that beauty is due to your other efforts—what you eat and whether your body is free of toxins (see Key 1). Dr. Perricone's anti-inflammatory diet also addresses this issue. Food supplements—the powerful vitamins, hormone relaxin, and herbs—are a factor as well. People who take in what is delicious and good for them experience increased energy, radiant skin, and a change in chi.

As we have learned, finding ways to deal with stress is important too. Getting enough sleep helps, and I incorporate the *Tao of Music* (to provide better absorption of topical applications) into my skincare regimen. Ten to 20 minutes of listening brings my brain and skin to alpha frequency and lets my skin soaks up the nutrients of the cream that Sam and I put together.

I know that even if I do all these things, I will eventually have wrinkles on my face or bags under my eyes, that I will eventually be old. But I want to grow old well and wise, have fun with life, and not, like previous generations, live in the past.

Just a few minutes ago I cut out of the *New York Times Magazine* a feature story on five women ages 67 to 84 still contributing to the design industry. I'll frame their pictures and put them on the wall of my office to remind me that I too can lead a vital life, not disappear into the twilight zone. I admit I want to look youthful, but I also follow the *Tao of Youth* to be healthy and to avoid "acting old" as well. Dr. Erno Laszlo is right—you cannot have beauty without health. It's not one or the other.

To accomplish the balance of good health and beauty is work. Living in a higher consciousness takes effort too. I'm not saying you must do what I do—a lot of it may not even be right for you. You may take a different approach—if so, more power to you. I do say you should make your choices consciously. This path is not easy given the habits of our society at large. But the rewards of using the keys to the *Tao of Youth* far outpace the pain. Just know that these outside factors accelerate skin age:

- overexposure to the sun
- primary and secondary cigarette smoke
- environmental toxins
- poor diet
- excessive alcohol consumption
- stress
- harsh soap or detergent-based moisturizers
- sleep deprivation

Skincare products can help you to:

- repair free-radical damage through the use of antioxidant-active ingredients
- exfoliate through ingredients that help cells to regenerate like younger skin
- moisturize with water-based rather than oil-based ingredients
- balance hormones
- elasticize skin through ingredients that promote collagen production
- improve microcirculation of the capillaries to make you glow.

And remember that traditional Chinese physicians are able to read the health status of individuals in their skin and chi. Those around you, perhaps without knowing it, will do the same.

Wild Camellias and Soup

Wild Camellia-Seed Oil

Wild camellias grow widely in the northern part of China. They bloom in November and last for about a month. The seeds take about six months to ripen before they are ready to be picked. Each seed looks something like a chestnut. Some are roasted, and some are cold-pressed for their oil. In ancient times the oil was used to preserve the wood pillars of buildings such as Japanese temples.

My first memory of camellia-seed oil is of the residue sold in a compressed round cake that our family's household workers used to wash their hair. (The village women in rural areas use these cakes too.) The women had pitch black, shiny hair worn in long pigtails or tied up in buns. I loved to watch them as they sat in our courtyard during rest time, combing each other's hair.

If you travel through the regions that produce camellias, you will notice that the people there look young and healthy, that both men and women have smooth skin. Everyone there works with camellia-seed oil, applies it to the skin, and consumes it. Just like the Spaniards and Italians full of olive oil, these northern Chinese people benefit from their consumption of oleic acid, a main ingredient in camellia-seed oil.

The use of camellia-seed oil for skincare dates back 3,000 years to its peak during the Ming and Qing dynasties of China. According to early gossip, Empress Dowager Cixi of the Qing dynasty used camellia oil for massage and on her face, to keep her skin smooth and bright. Thanks to a missionary priest who introduced the oil to Europe, Josephine, mistress of Napoleon, also used it for her face and body. She planted camellias, harvested the seed, and pressed the oil for her own consumption. More recently, Soong Mei-ling Madame Chiang Kai-shek, when asked at age 100 about skincare, said she used camellia oil for face and body. Known for her poise, she was a political partner to her husband, sometimes appearing before the U.S. Congress to win support for China's efforts. I was always impressed by her intellect and beauty.

Japanese women have used this oil more than those in China or Hong Kong, where Western cosmetic companies have strong brand identification (Chanel, for example). You cannot convince women in Hong Kong to buy otherwise. They have the idea that unless you spend a lot of money, the cosmetics you buy will not be good. Modern marketing is powerful!

In Japan, however, to which camellia oil was first imported during the Tang dynasty, there is a camellia oil club (something like a Costco membership) in every city. Now the Japanese produce their own camellia-seed oil. Some major cosmetics companies use the oil as a base, but few market it as a stand-alone product.

Camellia-seed oil contains:

- oleic acid (82.3–86 percent, depending on whom you're talking to)
- linolenic acid (5 percent)
- palmitic acid (7.4 percent)
- unsaponifiable (unable to decompose) matter (0.9 percent)
- phytosterol (0.6 percent)
- other components including vitamins and proteins.

The Good Acid

Greece and Italy have been found to have the lowest number of deaths from heart disease, whereas the United States has the highest. The Harvard School of Public Health has suggested that women who ingest olive oil are 25 percent less likely to get breast cancer than women who don't. What's in olive oil that makes the difference? Oleic acid, providing powerful health benefits to all!

But wait! Wild-camellia-seed oil contains at least 82.3 percent oleic acid, olive oil only 65 percent. Known as the Chinese olive oil, camellia-seed oil is superior to olive oil in terms of its oleic acid content.

About Oleic Acid

Many studies have shown the healing properties of oleic acid—a member of the omega-9 family, a nonessential monounsaturated fatty acid. Oleic acid helps keep the membrane fluid of skin cells soft and stable. It helps the complexion through ingestion of topical applications. Oleic acid (and the ellagitannins found in camellia seed) decreases oxidation of the LDLs ("bad" cholesterol) that accompany aging.

In addition, Javier Menendez of the Northwestern University Feinberg School of Medicine in Chicago along with colleagues in the United States and Spain, has conducted studies showing that oleic acid suppresses the action of cancer cells (oncogenes) and improves the effectiveness of the breast-cancer drug Herceptin®.

Physicians and researchers have been aware that a Mediterranean diet reduces the risk of breast cancer and other illnesses such as heart disease for some time. But "We have something now that [explains] why the Mediterranean diet is so healthy," Menendez says. "Oleic acid, is able to down-regulate the most important oncogene in breast cancer . . . The most important source of oleic acid is olive oil."

The skincare functions of camellia oil:

- Smoothing rough skin, making it appear tighter and more elastic
- Lightening black and red spots
- Reversing damage due to exposure to sunlight
- Tightening pores of face and body.
- Reducing wrinkles and making skin glow
- Improving blotchy, dry, and scaly skin
- Moisturizing the skin

According to skincare experts in China and Japan, camellia-seed oil is the most easily absorbed plant oil for human skin. But you don't need an expert—I've tried many oils in a 30-second test. Camellia-seed oil is most quickly absorbed by hands and face. It penetrates the deep layers of the skin, making it soft, fresh, and elastic.

The flowers of camellia plants come in three different colors: white, pink, and golden yellow. Different colors grow in different parts of China. Some claim golden yellow is the best, and some think it's pink. Wild camellia-seed oil does seem to vary in purity; the more yellow, greasy-feeling oils seem to me to be of lesser quality. About 96 percent to 97 percent pure camellia-seed oil is like virgin olive oil, much more satisfactory than the less-pure oil.

I choose quality oil not by the color of the flowers but according to its lightness to the touch and how fast my skin absorbs it—that 30-second test. I have been using wild camellia-seed oil for more than three years to remove makeup before washing with the mild sea mud of the Lazlo regimen, and I love it.

Wild camellia-seed oil is even better than olive oil for eating and cooking. You can use it in salads and salad dressings, as well as in regular cooking—in all the ways you would use olive oil. Even better, camellia oil can be used for stir-frying, which you cannot do with olive oil because of its lower smoking (flashpoint) temperature. Wild camellia-seed oil tolerates higher temperature, making it ideal for cooking as well as for topical use. Use this oil quickly, whether for topical application or as part of your diet, because its shelf life (that is, the time before it becomes rancid) is only about two years.

Use wild camellia-seed oil in your cooking and eating, use it alone to cleanse your skin, and use our Biolaxin™ (relaxin) skin cream, which contains camellia-seed oil as well. These measures, combined with appropriate enzyme supplementation to aid digestion and an occasional healing and skin-enriching soup or drink (see opposite and following), build on the solid foundation of Keys 1–4, to ensure that your skin reflects a younger you.

If even that is not enough, check out "If You're Getting It Fixed," starting on page 159.

Healing Soups

In researching the healing soups that the Chinese have drunk for centuries, I found many ingredients known to help skin and hair. These recipes have been handed down from one generation to another, especially in the southern part of China where I grew up.

The use of certain herbs, through the experience of everyday persons as well as of wise Chinese physicians, has also been passed down to the modern day. You can find information on the subject in many Traditional Chinese Medicine (TCM) textbooks. The famous Li Shi-zhen's herb book *Ben Cao Gang Mu* or *The Great Pharmacopoeia,* mentioned earlier, was the first organized by herb and disease. About 400 years ago Li Shi-zhen spent 30 years traveling across China to document the diseases and herbal remedies. Most TCM physicians use this reference often.

I have read through many Chinese medicinal and herbal-soup cookbooks to find soups and drinks that nourish the skin. The herbs in them assist other functions of the body, too, but the ones presented here are the most effective for the skin. As mentioned earlier, the southern Chinese use these drinks and soups as a way to soothe the digestive system. When I drink these soups, my gastrointestinal tract is happy; it resonates with these soups.

When I was younger I was always in a hurry, but now I like having a time to relax. I do that when I am drinking Oolong tea or one of these soups. I turn on the *Tao of Music,* and when the weather is good I sit next to my orb of stones and enjoy the moment. My Shangri-La is right in my backyard. Life could not be better.

For the following soup recipes, use the method for soups described on page 40 in Key 1.

Lean Pork Soup with Goji, Black Dates, and Dried Longans

3 oz goji

6 black dates

1–2 shelled, dried longans (dragon-eyed fruit)

1 lb lean pork

3 slices ginger

15 cups water

salt

1. Scald the lean pork.
2. Set aside and rinse the other ingredients.
3. Bring the water to a boil in a clay pot.
4. Put all the other ingredients into the pot.
5. Cook over high heat 15-20 minutes.
6. Reduce to low heat and simmer 1–2 hours.
7. Season with salt and serve.

Your local co-op may carry goji under the name goji or wolfberries. Goji contain 300 times more antioxidants than oranges. Goji is known to help eyesight as well as to enhance the skin. Black dates differ from the red dates used in earlier recipes in this book; black dates are much sweeter and soothe the nerves.

Longan—my childhood favorite—is also called dragon-eyes fruit (the seeds look like the eyes of a dragon). Longan and lichi (or lychee) are in season about the same time. I can eat a lot of longan with no problem, but I get a rash if I each too much lichi. Both promote blood-cell formation, energize chi, and nourish the organs.

Fujian, the town my family came from, is famous for its longan. If a mother was unable to produce enough milk for her baby, the villagers cooked dried longan with rice as a supplement.

Chicken with He Shou Wu, Fu Ling, and Bai Zhu

5 oz he shou wu

2–3 ounces fu ling

1 oz bai zhu

1 free-range chicken

15 cups water

2 slices ginger

1. Scald chicken.
2. Rinse and cut chicken into halves or quarters depending on the size or shape of your pot.
3. Rinse the other ingredients.
4. Bring the water to a boil, then add the other ingredients and boil for 15–20 minutes.
5. Reduce heat to low and simmer 2 hours.
6. Add salt and serve.

The herbs in this soup promote blood-cell formation, improve the texture of the skin, and energize chi. Adjust the ingredient (herbs and water) according to your taste. If you are curious, buy a Chinese-herb soup book and experiment a little. The taste of this soup is strong and may take some getting used to. A smaller amount of herbs provides a milder taste. My brother Sam likes only the preceding recipe.

Drinks for Improving Your Skin

Ground Walnut and Almond Drink

1 tsp ground walnut
1 tsp ground almond
1 tsp honey
Warm water to taste

1. Mix the ground walnut and almond with honey.
2. Add sufficient warm water.

This drink improves skin texture and strengthens the liver and brain.

————————

Ground Almond and Black Sesame Seed Drink

1½ tsp ground almond
1½ tsp ground black sesame seed
½ cup soymilk
1 cup Rice Dream
Honey to taste

1. Mix ground almond and black sesame seed together with the two kinds of milk.
2. Add honey or other sweetener to taste.
3. Drink this twice a day to help prevent discoloration of your skin. (It takes awhile to see the difference.)

Assorted Rice Soup

1 cup red rice

1 cup brown rice

1 cup wild rice

15 cups of water

1. Rinse all the rice.
2. Bring water to a boil and add all the rice.
3. Cook over high heat 20 minutes.
4. Reduce heat to low heat and simmer for 20 minutes.
5. Add honey to taste.
6. Eat 8 oz once a day and refrigerate what is left for another day.

This soup—rich in amino acids, vitamins, and minerals—boosts the vitality and beauty of your skin. Eat the rice, too!

———

Black Dates in Wine

1 lb black dates

1 bottle Old Shaoxing wine (20 oz)

Sealed glass bottle

1. Rinse black dates and leave them to dry to touch.
2. Put wine and black dates into a glass bottle and seal it.
3. Open after three months.
4. Separate wine and black dates and store them in separate jars. Adjust the proportion of wine to dates in each jar according to taste.
5. Drink in moderation to maintain good health and youthful energy.

Ching-Po-Leung and Egg Dessert Soup

This nutritious dessert, particularly for vegetarians who eat eggs, provides high-quality protein. Vegans can skip the egg and use more dried bean curd. *The New York Times* introduced ching-po-leung in a recent Sunday edition.

> 1 package ching-po-leung
> 4 oz dried bean curd
> 6 slabs raw brown sugar (Chinese brown sugar comes in slabs)
> 12 cups water

1. Rinse ching-po-leung ingredients and dried bean curd separately.
2. Bring water to boil.
3. Put all ingredients except eggs, into the pot.
4. Cook 15 minutes over high heat.
5. Reduce to low heat and simmer 1 hour.
6. Add hard-boiled eggs and boil for another 5 minutes.
7. Eat all the soup, including the solid ingredients.

Ching-po-leung is a prepackaged collection of ingredients including sha shen, yu zhu, lotus seeds, lily bulb, fox nuts, huai shan, and pearl barley or Job's tears, available at any Chinese grocery store. Chinese people eat it on hot, humid days to rid the body of Heat and Dampness. The other herbs improve the overall health of your inner skin as reflected in your outside skin: Yu zhu nourishes yin, strengthens lungs, and improves skin texture. Lily bulb calms nerves and energizes chi. Lotus seeds strengthen the heart, liver, spleen, and kidney and promote blood-cell formation. Dried bean curd provides protein. My friend Christine advises me when my voice sounds raspy after travel to make soup with yu zhu to clear my throat and lungs. After I drink such a soup (I add goji and lily bulbs), my voice regains its clarity.

If You're Getting It Fixed

Many women attending our workshops have asked my brother Sam about preparing themselves for plastic surgery. Here are his suggestions for what to do both before and after surgery:

The best preparation for plastic surgery involves paying attention to two areas we've already discussed—the reduction of water weight and the activity of relaxin in the skin. As mentioned earlier, I have found that many patients in surgery show evidence of lymphedema—or water within the interstitial spaces from partial blockage of the lymphatic systems (see Key 1). This water weight impedes the outcome and impacts the recovery time of surgery, particularly in regard to infection and post-surgical swelling. Surgeons seldom focus on this aspect of care, but if you prepare adequately, you can decrease your chances of infection, reduce swelling, heal faster, and recover more quickly from plastic surgery.

Surgery, particularly that involving the superficial skin, greatly disrupts the lymphatic flow important to draining fluid from the interstitial space to the lymph glands and eventually back to the systemic circulation. Sometimes surgery in the lower abdomen or lower back disrupts lymphatic drainage enough to swell one leg more than the other. This is common in patients with multiple back or abdominal surgeries. So, for minimal invasion, fast healing, and at least symmetrical rather than asymmetrical drainage, attend to your lymphatic system in preparation for plastic surgery.

Why plastic surgery in particular? Plastic surgery involves only the superficial layers of the skin, disrupting lymphatic drainage to such a degree that if it involves just one side of the body, the difference in drainage will vary enough to make a difference in swelling highly visible. Patients with breast augmentation, for instance, may find some time after the surgery that one part is bigger than the other. This is related to the disruption of lymphatic drainage—one area draining more slowly than the other. Wearing a too-tight bra also affects lymphatic drainage, sometimes pushing the breast prematurely into a different size or shape.

How does this apply to the plastic surgeries of the face? A facelift may appear to work well for some time. But think of the faces of the aging celebrities who have had multiple facelifts. As they age, their faces become lumpy. Certain areas are a bit bigger and lumpier on one side than on the other. The face is and appears to be asymmetrical. The difference may be subtle, but it is definitely noticeable. This is the result of disrupted and varying lymphatic drainage after surgery. Once a person has a lymphatic change due to surgery and begins to gain weight (particularly to gain net water weight), she almost always shows varied swelling along the edges of past surgical sites.

How can one avoid this problem? First, keep any invasive procedure as minimal as possible. Delay major surgery, such as an entire facelift, which disrupts almost the entire facial lymphatic drainage. Second, prepare for your surgery by draining as much lymphatic water as possible from your body and your face. This gives your surgeon a way to estimate more accurately and thus accomplish surgical and sculptural symmetry so that the lymphatic drainage is symmetrical too.

Not only is lymphatic drainage (getting rid of the water weight) important to the surgeon producing an attractive outcome, it also affects the healing of the surgical site. The extra water within a person's body drains toward the disrupted area, causing the incision to heal at a slower rate than normal. Also the area is prone to infection, which may cause other disruptions, depending on the particular site.

What about relaxin? Good-quality collagen (relaxin's cell-renewal activity, see Key 2) is a must for the healing of plastic surgery to produce a good result. Relaxin increases microcirculation in all the organs, including the skin. It helps regulate collagen production, which speeds healing, and produces a more elastic collagen, which results in reduced and better scar formation. Attention to your body's capacity for cell regeneration is the other side of the plastic surgery coin.

For the best overall surgical experience, recovery, and result, prepare for plastic surgery in these ways:

- Drain as much extra lymphatic water from your body as possible so that the surgery and drainage are symmetrical. (See Key 1.)

- Take Biolaxin™ (relaxin) for several months before the surgery for increased microcirculation and quick healing.
- After surgery, apply relaxin cream to the incision site to minimize scarring.

The no-gluten and no-casein diet is important both before and after your operation. Adherence to a no-gluten diet minimizes lymphatic swelling for minimal water weight gain. The weight gain after surgery initially consists of water weight, not fat. Fat weight usually increases in an overall manner, whereas lymphatic water weight gain may distort the surgical result—causing lumpiness of the face or asymmetrical enlargement of the breasts or abdomen. The no-gluten diet thus will extend from five to ten years the aesthetic result of your surgery. Of course, we cannot rely on plastic surgery to "fix" everything that might make us appear older. The best preparation for plastic surgery is a healthy lifestyle—healthy eating, balanced hormones, regular exercise to maintain muscle tone, and a calm and serene outlook—the *Tao of Youth*.

Follow these steps for healthy, younger-looking skin. Clear, youthful skin reflects how healthy you are. There is no magic potion to erase wrinkles, but if you follow these steps you can have radiant skin. Having that glow is more important than worrying about wrinkles. A healthy aura or chi radiates vitality: a few wrinkles merely show experience—your laughing, your crying, your wisdom.

1. Feed your skin. Use the *Tao of Youth* eating strategy to provide a lot of antioxidants and to flush undigested proteins from your lymphatic system. That will quickly result in fresh and glowing skin. If you avoid gluten and casein, you will eat a lot of food full of nutrients such as those in Dr. Perricone's anti-inflammatory diet (though he does not address the hard-to-digest foods). Follow a good, high-dose multivitamin and mineral regimen according to the recommendations of such as Julian Whitaker (Forward Plus) or Garry Gordon (Beyond Chelation). Most of them also include omega-3 and -6. A tablespoon or two daily of flaxseed oil or ground flaxseed will do wonders for your skin.

2. Shield against UV radiation. Protect yourself from exposure to ultraviolet radiation from sunlight. For everyday protection use a sunscreen with an SPF of at least 15. For prolonged exposure, always use a sun block.

3. Avoid smoking. People who smoke a lot have skin similar to that exposed to UV radiation from sunlight. Studies show smoking and UV radiation have the same effect. If possible, stop smoking.

4. Drink plenty of water: Seventy percent of the dermis, or inner layer of the skin, is water. One of the main reasons that your skin sags and wrinkles as you age is that the dermis loses about 30 percent of its total water content along the way. Hydrate your skin from the inside by drinking a good amount of purified water.

5. Help your skin glow. Collagen is the most important supporting structure for your skin. The skin of women who are pregnant glows partly because they produce ten times the normal amount of estrogen, progesterone, and relaxin. The microcirculation of their blood vessels is well-tuned. Keep your hormones in balance with a good HRT program. A good topical cream containing vitamin C helps too.

6. Find a good skincare regimen. Find a cleansing program right for your skin type and an appropriate night cream. Sam's Biolaxin™ (relaxin) cream has worked wonders for many women. Many mention noticing a new glow.

7. Find ways to reduce stress. Allow yourself to be as calm as possible; be able to relax so your skin can absorb more moisture. Listening to special-frequency music as you apply your skin products will provide maximum absorption (see Galvanic Skin Responce on page 125).

8. Get adequate sleep. Ward Dean says you age rapidly if you don't maintain a good sleep-wake cycle. Many pilots and flight attendants complain that the frequent disruption of their cycles causes them to "age before my eyes." This shows especially in their skin as compared with those who keep a normal schedule. A decrease in melatonin production as you age can also cause poor sleep. Supplementing with melatonin and/or relaxin helps restore deep, restful sleep.

You cannot stop aging, but you can make the best of it. Your skin is the first sign of how you care for the inside of your body. The *Tao of Youth* lifestyle is a continuum of care, a circle affecting and depending upon digestion, weight, hormone balance, musculoskeletal health, serenity, and the health of your skin. My brother, my sister, and I have discovered and implemented the *Tao of Youth*, thanks to our own questions and to Sam's treatment and observations of fibromyalgia patients for 20 years. We hope you find these discoveries to be useful and that you share your own discoveries with the world.

Conclusion

The Path

The book of Lao Tze—*Tao Tse Ching*—makes more sense to me than that of Confucius, who equates women with children and considers both to be ignorant. But the first poem of *Tao Tse Ching*—"The Path"—is difficult, especially for a young person. Lao Tse speaks without dogma, writes about nature and flow. As a teenager, I read it as so much mumbo-jumbo. Then one day I came across a book interpreting his poem. The explanation stays with me:

In ancient time, people walked with their bare feet to create a way. The way had a beginning and an end. But there were many paths—the usual and the unusual, the well trod and the untrod, the short-term and the long-term, the uphill and the downhill, and many more.

To illustrate: A horse grazing in the meadow somehow loses his way into the desert. He is hungry and thirsty. How can he save himself? Here are the options:

1. Take the usual path—continue and eventually die of exhaustion or thirst.
2. Take the unusual path—three more choices:
   - Backtrack to the meadow, with a 50/50 chance of making it.
   - Use every bit of strength to go through the desert as quickly as possible, with a 1 percent chance of survival.
   - Rest, listen for the direction of the wind, look for an animal, and drink its blood or follow it to water, with a 90 percent chance of success.

The wise horse, lost in the desert, follows the camel.

You must use what you know to find your own best path—even if you have to change or do the unfamiliar. Sometimes you see something and it means nothing; sometimes you see nothing and it means something. Life is full of mystery. Only you can discover and follow the path that is right for you.

The wise person, like the wise horse, is adaptable and resourceful—and thinks about what is possible and probable. Nothing is 100 percent certain—but do look for probabilities in your favor.

Our search for wellness and health has not followed the usual path. We have taken twists and turns, followed the best odds, taken byways and backtracked, sometimes found treasure, sometimes adapted it. This is the result—what has worked best for us. We hope it helps you find the best way for you.

Appendix: I Ching

Chinese people use *I Ching*, or *The Book of Changes*, the oldest classic text, to make predictions. *I Ching* is generally regarded as a product of Taoism. Use of *I Ching* often leads to uncannily accurate prediction. The sages of ancient China who compiled this system had knowledge not possessed by even the most learned men in the West.

The legendary sage Fuxi, who apparently lived about 7,000 years ago, is said to have developed the eight trigrams, or Pa Kua—the mystic symbols used in divination (Prediction). Among those using I Ching were Japanese military and naval commanders in World War II—Mao Zedong and Gen. Chiang Kai-shek—and German mathematician and philosopher Gottfried Wilhelm von Leibniz.

The exact process of *I Ching* is beyond human comprehension. It is the manifestation of an ultimate reality; its compilers seem to have been divinely inspired. It does provide practical results. By clever suggestion, *I Ching* prompts its users to retrieve information buried in the subconscious, often revealing great truths. It is not a book of magic spells but a retrieval system with mathematical precision.

Swiss psychologist Carl G. Jung explained the function of *I Ching* by what he called the "Law of Synchronicity," suggesting that similar events occur at one and the same time throughout the universe and to some degree influence each other. For instance, many people may at one time experience the feeling—a kind of sixth-sense reaction—that something is not right.

The people who put *I Ching* together probably made effective use of autosuggestion, retrieving information contained in their own subconscious that provided answers to their questions. Prompted by a single word, perhaps, a whole train of thought follows, setting their course.

Sources & resources

Introduction

I Ching (Book of Changes). James Legge's translation is available online at www.sacred-texts.com/ich/index.htm.

Lao Tze. *Tao Tse Ching.* Spellings of this and following ancient authors' names and titles vary. Peter H. Merel's translation of all 81 sections is available online at www.chinapage.com/gnl.html.

Sunzi. *Art of War.* Lionel Giles's translation is available at www.gutenberg.org/etext/132.

Key 1

The recipes in Key 1 are adapted by the author from family and traditional collections and from Chinese cookbooks not translated to English.

Diamond, Marilyn, and Donald Burton Schnell. *Fitonics™ for Life.* New York: Avon/Harper Collins, 1996.

Li, Shi-zhen. *Chinese Medicinal Herbs.* Trans. Smith F. Porter, ed. G. A. Stuart and Smith F. Porter. New York: Dover, 2003. This is a translation of the herbal section of *Ben Cao Gang Mu (The Great Pharmacopoeia).*

Lin, Luke (Lin, Kuang Chang). *Fresh, Light, Toxin-free.* Taiwan: Shy Mau, 2005.

Mok, Tin Chi. *Nutritious Soups for My Dearest Karen.* Beijing: China Light Industry Press, 2006.

Pitchford, Paul. *Healing with Whole Foods: Asian Traditions and Modern Nutrition* (3rd ed.). Berkeley, CA: North Atlantic Books, 2002.

Whitaker, Julian. *Health and Healing.* Subscribe to this newsletter at www.drwhitaker.com.

Whitaker, Julian, and Carol Colman. *Shed 10 Years in 10 Weeks.* Simon & Schuster: 1999.

Whitaker, Julian, and Michael T. Murray. *Dr. Whitaker's Guide to Natural Healing.* New York: Three Rivers Press, 1996.

Whitaker, Julian, and Peggy Dace. *The Memory Solution: Dr. Julian Whitaker's 10-Step Program to Optimize Your Memory and Brain Function.* Garden City Park, NY: Avery, 2002.

Yen, Kun-ying. *The Illustrated Chinese Materia Medica: Crude and Prepared Drugs*. Taipei: SMC, 1995.

Key 2

For studies on the hormone relaxin, see Selected Studies on Effects of Relaxin following this more general reference list.

Chauchard, Claude. *Live Longer, Live Better: The Life-Capital Method*. Paris: Encre/Hong Kong: N.p. (Chinese edition), 1996, 1998, 2006.

Dean, Ward. "Neuroendocrine Theory of Aging." (Series of special reports in) *Vitamin Research News* (a food supplement newsletter), 1999.

Dilman, V. M., and John Wright. *The Law of Deviation of Homeostasis and Diseases of Aging*. N.c.: N.p., 1981. Ward Dean refers to and summarizes Dilman and Wright's work in "Neuroendocrine Theory of Aging," *Vitamin Research Products*, found at http://www.vrp.com.

Gittleman, Anne Louise. *Super Nutrition for Menopause: Take Control of Your Life Now and Enjoy New Vitality*. New York: Pocket Books, 1998.

———. *Super Nutrition for Women: A Food-wise Guide for Health, Beauty, Energy, and Immunity*. New York: Bantam (reissue), 1997.

Ivell, Richard. "This Relaxin Is Relaxing Too Long." *Science* 295 (no. 555, January 2002): 637–38.

Kurzweil, Kurt. *Fantastic Voyage*. Toronto: Penguin Group, 2005.

Lark, Susan. *The Menopause Self Help Book: A Woman's Guide to Feeling Wonderful for the Second Half of Her Life*. (4th ed.) Berkeley, CA: Celestial Arts, 1990. For Lark's newsletter, *Women Wellness Today*, see www.drlark.com.

Lark, Susan, and James A. Richards. *The Chemistry of Success: Six Secrets of Peak Performance*. San Jose, CA: Bay Books, 1999.

Lee, John R., Jesse Hanley, and Virginia Hopkins. *What Your Doctor May Not Tell You about Premenopause: Balance Your Hormones and Your Life from Thirty to Fifty*. New York: Warner Wellness, 1999.

Life Extension Foundation. *Disease Prevention and Treatment* (4th ed). Fort Lauderdale, FL: Life Extension Media, 2003.

Loes, Michael. The Aspirin Alternative: *The Natural Way to Overcome Chronic Pain, Reduce Inflammation and Enhance the Healing Process*. Topanga, CA: Freedom Press, 1999.

———. *The Healing Response: Applying the Ten Principles and Laws of Healing*. Topanga, CA: Freedom Press, 2003.

Marchione, Marilynn. "Dramatic Decline in Breast Cancer." *Minneapolis Star Tribune,* December 15, 2006.

Northrup, Christine. *The Wisdom of Menopause.* New York: Bantam, 2001

Parker, William H. *A Gynecologist's Second Opinion: The Questions and Answers You Need to Take Charge of Your Health.* East Rutherford, NJ: Plume (Penguin), 2002.

Parker, William H., Amy Roseman, and Rachel Parker. *The Incontinence Solution: Answers for Women of All Ages.* New York: Fireside (Simon & Schuster), 2002.

Parker, William H., et al. "Ovarian Conservation at the Time of Hysterectomy for Benign Disease." *Journal of Obstetrics and Gynecology* 106 (August 2005): 219–26.

Roizen, Michael F. *The RealAge® Makeover: Take Years off Your Looks and Add Them to Your Life.* New York: HarperCollins, 2004.

Seaman, Barbara, "Keeping All Your Eggs in Your Basket." *O, the Oprah Magazine* (October 2006).

Somers, Suzanne. *Ageless.* New York: Crown, 2006.

——. *The Sexy Years.* New York: Crown, 2004.

Wright, Jonathan V. *Natural Hormone Replacement.* Petaluma, CA: Smart Publications, 1997.

——. *Nutrition & Healing* (newsletter). Subscription information at www.wrightnewsletter. com. Free *Library of Food and Vitamin Cures* includes *New Secrets Every Woman Needs to Know.*

Key 3

Brody, Jane E. "To Avoid 'Boomeritis.' Exercise, Exercise, Exercise." *New York Times,* December 20, 2006.

Lark, Susan. *Women Wellness Today* (newsletter). See www.drlark.com.

Lerner, Barron H. "No Shrinking Violet: Rose Kushner and the Rise of American Breast Cancer Activism." *Western Journal of Medicine* 174 (no. 5, May 2001): 362–65.

Li, Shi-zhen. *Chinese Medicinal Herbs.* Trans. Smith F. Porter, ed. G. A. Stuart and Smith F. Porter. New York: Dover, 2003. This is a translation of the herbal section of *Ben Cao Gang Mu (The Great Pharmacopoeia).*

Parker, William H., et al. "Ovarian Conservation at the Time of Hysterectomy for Benign Disease." *Journal of Obstetrics and Gynecology* 106 (August 2005): 219–26.

Sellmeyer Deborah E., et al., for the Study of Osteoporotic Fractures Research Group. "A High Ratio of Dietary Animal to Vegetable Protein Increases the Rate of Bone Loss and the Risk of Fracture in Postmenopausal Women." *American Journal of Clinical Nutrition* 73 (no. 1, January 2001): 118–22.

Tan, Amy. *Joy Luck Club.* New York: Penguin, 1989. (Many other editions are available.)

———. *The Kitchen God's Wife.* New York: Ballantine, 1991.

Whitaker, Julian. *Health and Healing.* See www.drwhitaker.com.

Williams, David. "Better Bone-Builder and More Lifesavers for Women." *Alternatives for the Health-Conscious Individuals,* 2006.

Key 4

Alder, Vera Stanley. *The Finding of the Third Eye.* Boston: Weiser Books, 1970 (and subsequent editions).

Anderson, James W., and Maury M. Breecher. *Live Longer Better: Dr. Anderson's Complete Antiaging Health Program.* New York: Carroll & Graf Publishers, 1997). This book mentions the work of James Heffley, a nutritionist who writes "To Your Health," a regular column for the *Austin (Texas) Chronicle.*

Apter, Michael J. *Reversal Theory: The Dynamics of Motivation, Emotion and Personality.* (2nd ed.) Oxford, England: Oneworld, 2007.

Bateman, Wesley H. Browse websites for RA music/Batemen and you will find, for example, his "Law of Sympathetic Resonance," part of *Nefer's House of Cosmic Harmony & RA Math Lesson 6.* See www.geocities.com/CapeCanaveral/Hall/3324/nefershouse.htm.

Bliokh, P. V., et al. *The Schumann Resonances in the Earth-Ionosphere Cavity* (IEE Electromagnetic Waves Series, vol. 9). London: Peter Peregrinus, 1980.

Brown, Dan. *The Da Vinci Code.* New York: Doubleday, 2003 (and subsequent editions).

Dalai Lama and Howard C. Cutler. *The Art of Happiness.* New York: Riverhead Books, 1998.

Dalai Lama and Jeffrey Hopkins. *How to Expand Love.* New York: Atria (Simon & Schuster), 2005.

———. *How to Practice the Way to a Meaningful Life.* New York: Pockets Books, 2002.

Freud, Sigmund. The wikipedia.com entry for Freud is documented and contains a synopsis of his work. There are many other sources on his work.

Godwin, Malcolm. *The Holy Grail: It Origins, Secrets and Meaning Revealed.* London: Labyrinth, 1994.

MacLaine, Shirley. *The Camino: A Journey of the Spirit.* Pocket Books 2000.

———. *Dancing While You Can.* New York: Bantam, 1991.

———. *It's All in the Playing.* New York: Bantam, 1988.

Mathison, Volney. *Secret Power of the Crystal Pendulum.* N.c.: N.p., 1954. Complete publishing information is unknown, but descriptions of Mathison and his work are available online.

Osho, Bhagwan Shree Rajneesh. *The Sound of Silence: The Diamond in the Lotus.* Cologne, West Germany: Rebel, 1989.

———. *Tao: The Golden Gate.* Oregon: Acharaya Rajneesh Foundation International, 1984. Available online at oshoworld.com/onlinebooks.

Redfield, James, and Carol Adrienne. *The Celestine Prophecy: An Experiential Guide.* New York: Warner Books, 1995.

Trungpa, Chogyam. *Meditation in Action.* Boston: Shambhala, 1996.

———. *Shambhala: Sacred Path of the Warrior.* Boston: Shambhala, Boston 1988.

Weil, Andrew. *Spontaneous Healing: How to Discover and Enhance Your Body's Natural Ability to Maintain and Heal Itself.* New York: Ballantine Group, 1996 (reprint edition).

Williamson, Marianne. *Everyday Grace, Having Hope, Finding Forgiveness, and Making Miracles.* New York: Riverhead Books, 2002.

———. *The Gift of Change.* San Francisco: Harper, 2004.

———. *Illuminata.* New York: Random House, 1994.

———. *Return to Love: Reflections on the Principles of "A Course in Miracles."* New York: Harper, 1996 (reissue).

Key 5

The author translated the history of and information about wild camellia-seed oil from a Chinese book by Sheng Wen. The recipes in Key 5 were adapted from family and traditional collections and from Chinese cookbooks not translated to English.

Dilman, Vladimir, and Ward Dean. *The Neuroendocrine Theory of Aging and Degenerative Disease.* Pensacola, FL: Center for Bio-Gerontology, 1992.

Jewell, Diana Lewis. *The Angel of Beauty: The Story of Dr. Erno Laszlo.* New York: Erno Laszlo LLC, 1998.

Menendez, Javier, et al. "Oleic Acid, the Main Monounsaturated Fatty Acid of Olive Oil, Suppresses Her-2/Neu (Erbb-2) Expression and Synergistically Enhances the Growth Inhibitory Effects of Trastuzumab (Herceptin™) in Breast Cancer Cells with Her-2/Neu Oncogene Amplification." *Annals of Oncology* 16 (January 2005): 359–71. Reports of the findings also appear on websites such as News-Medical.Net.

New York Times Style Magazine, October 8, 2006.

Perricone, Nicholas. *The Perricone Prescription.* New York: Harper Resource, 2002.

———. *The Perricone Promise.* New York: Warner Books, 2004.

Swerdlow, Joel L. "Unmasking Skin." *National Geographic* (November 2002): 36–63.

Conclusion

Lao Tze. *Tao Tse Ching*. Spellings of this and following ancient authors' names and titles vary. Peter H. Merel's translation of all 81 sections is available online at <u>www.chinapage.com/gnl.html.</u>

Appendix

I Ching (Book of Changes). James Legge's translation is available online at <u>www.sacred-texts.com/ich/index.htm.</u>

Jung, Carl. The <u>www.wikipedia.com</u> entry for Carl Jung includes an extensive bibliography of his works and a list of works about him.

Selected Articles on Effects of Relaxin

These are just a few of the dozens of scientific studies and articles on the functions and effects of relaxin. The citations for the following, most recent studies are in standard rather than scientific form for the benefit of the general reader. Abstracts and/or full text of all the following are available on the Internet. Just type the title of the article into your browser.

Review

Bani, D. "Relaxin: A Pleiotropic Hormone." *General Pharmacology* 28 (no. 1, January 1997): 13–22.

Geddes, B. J., and A. J. Summerlee. "The Emerging Concept of Relaxin as a Centrally Acting Peptide Hormone with Hemodynamic Actions." *Journal of Neuroendocrinology* 7 (no. 6, June 1995): 411–17.

Binding Site

Kohsaka, T., et al. "Identification of Specific Relaxin-Binding Cells in the Human Female. *Biology of Reproduction* 59 (no. 4, October 1998): 991–99.

Cancer Issues

Bigazzi, M., et al. "Relaxin Influences the Growth of MCF-7 Breast Cancer Cells. Mitogenic and Antimitgenic Action Depends on Peptide Concentration." *Cancer* 70 (no. 3, August 1992): 639–43.

Norrby, K., et al. "Relaxin, a Potent Microcirculatory Effector, Is Not Angiogenic." *International Journal of Microcirculation, Clinical and Experimental* 16 (no. 5, September-October 1996): 227–31.

Sacchi, T. B., et al. "Relaxin Influences Growth, Differentiation and Cell-Cell Adhesion of Human Breast-Cancer Cells in Culture." *International Journal of Cancer* 57 (no. 1, April 1994): 129–34.

Collagen

Huang, C., et al. "Stimulation of Collagen Secretion by Relaxin and Effect of Oestrogen on Relaxin Binding in Uterine Cervical Cells of Pigs." *Journal of Reproduction and Fertility* 98 (no. 1, May 1993): 153–58.

Kibblewhite, D., et al. "The Effect of Relaxin on Tissue Expansion." *Archives of Otolaryngology—Head and Neck Surgery* 118 (no. 2, February 1992): 153–56.

Parsell, D. A., et al. "Relaxin Binds to and Elicits a Response from Cells of the Human Monocytic Cell Line, THP-1." *Journal of Biological Chemistry* 271 (no. 44, November 1, 1996): 27936–41.

Unemori, E. N., and E. P. Amento. "Relaxin Modulates Synthesis and Secretion of Procollagenase and Collagen by Human Dermal Fibroblasts." *Journal of Biological Chemistry* 265 (no. 18 June 25, 1995): 10681–85.

Insulin-like Growth Factor, Prolactin, Growth Hormone

Bethea, C. L., et al. "The Effect of Relaxin Infusion on Prolactin and Growth Hormone Secretion in Monkeys." *Journal of Clinical Endocrinology and Metabolism* 69 (no. 5, November 1989): 956–62.

Ohleth, K. M., and C. A. Bagnell. "Relaxin-Induced Deoxyribonucleic Acid Synthesis in Porcine Granulosa Cells Is Mediated by Insulin-Like Growth Factor-I." *Biology of Reproduction* 53 (no. 6, December 1995): 1286–92.

Sortino. M. A., et al. "Relaxin Stimulates Prolactin Secretion from Anterior Pituitary Cells." *Endocrinology* 124 (April 1989): 2013–14.

Nitric Oxide Pathway

Bani, D., et al. "Relaxin Activates the L-Arginine-Nitric Oxide Pathway in Vascular Smooth Muscle Cells in Culture." *Hypertension* 31 (no. 6, June 1998): 1240-47.

Bani-Sacchi, T., et al. "Relaxin-Induced Increased Coronary Flow through Stimulation of Nitric Oxide Production." *British Journal of Pharmacology* 116 (no. 1, September 1995): 1589–94

Masini, E. "Relaxin Inhibits Histamine Release from Mast Cells: Involvement of Nitric Oxide Production." *Inflammation Research* 44 (April 1995, Supplement): S12–13.

Cardiovascular

Coulson, C. C., et al. "Central Hemodynamic Effects of Recombinant Relaxin in the Isolated, Perfused Rat Heart Model." *Obstetrics & Gynecology* 87 (April 1996): 610–12.

Di Bello, M. G., et al. "Relaxin Enhances the Coronary Outflow in Perfused Guinea-Pig Heart: Correlation with Histamine and Nitric Oxide." *Inflammatory Research* 44 (April 1995, Supplement 1): S102–03.

Masini, E., et al. "The Effect of Relaxin on Myocardial Ischaemia-Reperfusion Injury and Histamine Release in Vitro and in Vivo." *Inflammation Research* 45 (March 1996, Supplement 1): S27–28.

Parry, L. J., et al. "The Cardiovascular Effects of Porcine Relaxin in Brattleboro Rats." *Endocrine* 8 (no. 3, June 1998): 317–22.

Taylor, M. J., and C. L. Clark. "Evidence for a Novel Source of Relaxin: Atrial Cardiocytes." *Journal of Endocrinology* 143 (no. 2, November 1994): R5–8.

Ward, D. G., et al. "Relaxin Increases Rat Heart Rate by a Direct Action on the Cardiac Atrium." *Biochemical and Biophysical Research Communications* 186 (no. 2, July 31, 1992): 999–1005.

Yang, R. H., et al. "Pressor and Bradycardic Effects of Centrally Administered Relaxin in Conscious Rats." *American Journal of Hypertension* 8 (no. 4, April 1995, Part 1): 375–81.

Insulin Binding

Olefsky J. M., et al. "Potentiation of Insulin Binding and Insulin Action by Purified Porcine Relaxin." *Annals of the New York Academy of Sciences* 380 (1982): 200–16.

Studies of Relaxin with Human Subjects

Some but not all of the following studies are available on the Internet; many were written before such studies were broadcast online and are not available there. Physicians are the most likely to have access, so they are presented in scientific form, in chronological order.

Treatment of the dysmenorrhea symptom complex: a preliminary report on the efficacy of a uterine-relaxing factor. (Jones GS: Am J Obst & Gynec. 67:628, March 1954)

Effects of administration of relaxin to human subjects. (Perkoff GT, et al.: J Clin Endocrinol. 14:531-539, May 1954)

Use of relaxin in treatment of threatened premature labor. (Abramson D; Reid DE: J Clin Endocrinol. 15: 206-209, Feb 1955)

Relaxin, the third ovarian hormone: Its experimental use in women. (Eichner E; Waltner C; Goodman M; Post S: Am J Obst & Gynec. 71: 1035-1048, May 1956)

Clinical evaluation of relaxin. (Folsome CE; Harami T; Lavietes SR; Massell GM: Obst & Gynec. 8: 536-544, Nov 1956)

The hormone relaxin in labor: Tocometric studies of effect on uterine contractions at term. (Kelly JV; Posse N: Obst & Gynec. 8: 531-535, Nov 1956)

A study of the effect of relaxin on contractility of the nonpregnant uterus by internal tocometry. (Posse N; Kelly JV: Surg Gynec & Obst. 103: 687-694, Dec 1956)

Preliminary report on the use of relaxin in the management of threatened premature labor. (McCarthy JJ Jr; Erving HW; Laufe LE: Am J Obstet & Gynec 74:134-8, July 1957)

Facilitation of full-term labor with relaxin. (Eisenberg L: JAOA 57:146-8, Oct 57)

Refined relaxin and length of labor: a preliminary report. (Birnberg CH; Abitbol MM: Obstet & Gynec 10:366-70, Oct 1957)

Use of relaxin in the treatment of scleroderma. (Casten GG, et al. JAMA 166:319, Jan 1958)

Relaxin: Its effects in a case of acrosclerosis. (Ismay G: Br J Dermatol: 70(5):171–175, May 1958)

Hormonal control of labor with relaxin and oxytocin. (Eisenberg L: JAOA 57:702-5, July 1958)

Some effects of relaxin in obstetrics. (Decker WH; Tthwaite W; Bordat S; Kayser R; Harami T; Campbell J: Obstet & Gynec 12:37-46, July 1958)

Effect of relaxin on normal labor. (Dill LV; Chanatry J: JAMA 167:1910-2, Aug 1958)

Primary dysmenorrhea: Treatment with relaxin. (Abramson D; Reid DE: Obst & Gynec 12:123-30, Aug 1958)

Use of relaxin in obstetrics. (Rothnem MS; Larson PN; Ingalls EG: Minnesota Medicine 544-6, Aug 1958)

Relaxin: A critical evaluation. (Stone ML; Sedlis A; Zuckerman M: Am J Obst & Gynec 76: 544-9, Sept 1958)

Oral Releasin in dysmenorrhea. (Crosley AP Jr; Thornton MJ; Campbell RE; Peckham B: J Clin Endroclinol Metab 18:1435-37, Dec 1958)

The effect of relaxin on the duration of labour induced by oxytocin. (Engstrom L; Wiqvist N: Acta Obstet Gynec Scand 38:172-80, 1959)

Effects of relaxin on the nonpregnant and pregnant uterus. (Kelly JV: Ann NY Acad Sci 75:998-1002, 9 Jan 1959)

Effects of relaxin on term and premature labor. (Stone ML; Sedlis A; Zuckerman MB: Ann NY Acad Sci 75:1011-5, 9 Jan 1959)

Relaxin in dysmenorrhea and its effect in vitro upon muscular contraction. (Kupperman HS; Rosenberg D; Cutler A: Ann NY Acad Sci 75:1003-10, 9 Jan 1959)

Some clinical observations of relaxin in obstetrics. (Decker WH: Ann NY Acad Sci 75:991-4, 9 Jan 1959)

Relaxin (Releasen) therapy in diffuse progressive scleroderma: a preliminary report. (Evans JA: AMA Arch Dermatol 79:64-72, Feb 1959)

Labor shortening devices: A study in relaxin and pitocin. (Rutherford RN; Banks AL; Coburn WA: Northwest Medicine p.389-92, March 1959)

Reaction to Cervilaxin: Report of a case. (Wendt WP; Wolfe CW: Obst & Gynec 13:574-5, May 1959)

Term labour: its facilitation by relaxin: a preliminary report. (Sands RX; Ko JH: Canad MAJ 80:886-90, 1 June 1959)

Relaxin: its effect on electively induced labor. (Babcock RJ; Peterson JH: Am J Obst & Gynec 78:33-37, July 1959)

The use of relaxin (Cervilaxin) in accelerating the first stage of labor. (Rothman ED; Bentley WG; Floyd WS: Am J Obst & Gynec 78: 38-41, July 1959)

Use of relaxin in management of ulceration and gangrene due to collagen disease. (Reynolds H; Livingwood CS: AMA Arch Derm 80:407-9, Oct 1959)

Relaxin in pulmonary fibrosis: Preliminary report. (Barthakur A; Bridges B; Harden KA: Med Ann DC 29:80-2, Feb 1960)

Behavior of the cervix during obstetric labor under the influence of relaxin. (Walczak JR: J Amer Osteopath Ass 59:649-52, Apr 60)

The use of relaxin in the management of the retained dead fetus. (Maclure JG; Ferguson JH: Amer J Obstet Gynec 79:801-4, Apr 1960)

Anaphylactic reaction to relaxin. (Levine RA; Kossmann RJ; Rogoff B: New Engl J Med 263:693-4, 6 Oct 1960)

A new approach to the management of obliterative peripheral arterial disease. (Casten GG; Gilmore HR; Houghton FE; Samuels SS: Angiology 11:408-14, Oct 1960)

Use of relaxin during parturition: Clinical observations. (Nesbitt RE Jr; Cirigliano G: New York J Med 61:90-7, 1 Jan 1961)

A study of relaxin in primigravidas. (Ware D; Hatnes DM: Amer J Obstet Gynec 83:792-4, 15 Mar 1962)

Connective tissue changes in the cervix during pregnancy and labor. (Buckingham JC; Selden R; Danfirth DN: Ann NY Acad Sci 97:733-42, 29 Sep 1962)

Clinical evaluation of relaxin in ulcerative ischemic vascular or collagen diseases. (Bradham GB; Stallworth JM; Brailsford LE; Threatt BA: Angiology 13:418-20, Sep 1962)

Relaxin in the treatment of localised scleroderma. (Wells RS: Trans St Johns Hosp Dermatol Soc 1963; 49: 149-51) [UI# 64073848]

Treatment of symphyseolysis with relaxin. (Jarvinen PA; Luukkainen T: Ann Chir Gynaec Fenn 52:251-4, 1963)

Hormonal influence in simple glaucoma: A preliminary report. (Paterson GD, et al. Brit J Ophal 47:129-37, Mar 1963)

The use of relaxin in progressive systemic sclerosis and other connective tissue diseases: A clinical study. (Rivelis AL, et al. Arch Interam Rheumatol; 28: 19-31, Mar-Jun 1965)

Ripening of the human cervix and induction of labour with purified porcine relaxin. (MacLennan AH; Lancet, 2 Feb 1980)

Cervical ripening with combinations of vaginal prostaglandin, F2-alpha estradiol, and relaxin. (MacLennan AH; Obstet Gynecol, Nov 1981)

Ripening of the human cervix with porcine ovarian relaxin. (Evans MI; Am J Obstet Gynecol, 15 Oct 1983)

The effect of porcine relaxin vaginally applied at human embryo transfer in an in vitro fertilization programme. (MacLennan AH; Aust N Z J Obstet Gynaecol, Feb 1985)

Ripening of the human cervix and induction of labor with intracervical purified porcine relaxin. (MacLennan AH; Obstet Gynecol, Nov 1986)

Resources

Alternative Medicine

American College for Advancement in Medicine (ACAM)
23121 Verdugo Drive, Suite 204
Laguna Hills, CA 92653
800-532-3688
www.acam.org

American Academy of Anti-aging Medicine
1510 West Montana Street
Chicago, IL 60614
773-528-4333
www.worldhealth.net

Life Extension
1100 West Commercial Blvd.
Fort Lauderdale, FL 33309
800-544-4440
www.lef.org.

(We recommend Life Extension memberships to most of our workshop attendees because in addition to the monthly magazine, LE has a wonderful published reference book called *Disease Prevention and Treatment.* LE also provides comprehensive hormone testing, offering complete male and female hormone panels.)

International Academy of Compound Pharmacists
P.O. Box 1365
Sugar Land, TX 77478
Phone: 281-933-8400
Toll-Free Referral Line 800-927-4227
www.iacprx.org

(Enter your zip code at this website to find a compound pharmacist in your area.)

Alternative Medicine Newsletters

Alternatives for the Health Conscious Individual (Dr. David Williams)
www.drdavidwilliams.com

Health and Healing: Your Definitive Guide to Wellness Medicine (Julian Whitaker, M.D.)
www.drwhitaker.com

Nutrition and Healing (Jonathan V. Wright, M.D.)
Subscription includes free Library of Nutritional Cures
www.wrightnewsletter.com

Women's Wellness Today (Susan Lark, M.D.)
www.drsusanlark.com

Heart, Health & Wellness: A Cardiologist's Guide to Total Wellness (Dr. Stephen Sinatra)
(Dr. Stephen Sinatra)
www.drsinatra.com

Food Supplement Sources

Most food supplements are available in food co-ops, natural-food stores, GNC, Whole food stores, drug stores, and many conventional groceries.

Internet Supplement Stores (a few examples)

www.swansonvitamins.com   www.iherb.com
www.prohealth.com   www.foryourhealth.com

For Mannatech producuts:
Anne Sween, Ph.D.
HealthMission
952-233-2208
annesween@mchsi.com
www.mannapages.com/annesween

Soup Ingredients and Herbs

Most Chinese soup ingredients and herbs are available in Asian grocery stores.

Pain Clinic

Samuel Yue, M.D.
Minnesota Pain Center
Elmo, MN
651-731-0707

Where to Get *Tao of Youth* Music and Biolaxin™ (Relaxin)
SKY Biohealth Solutions, Inc.*
10300 Valley View Road, Suite 107B
Eden Prairie, MN 55344
952-946-1550
Toll free: 1-888-946-1622
www.taoofyouth.com

* In the interests of full disclosure: two of the authors of this book, Sam Yue, M.D., and May Yue, own and are officers of SKY Biohealth Solutions, Inc. The following sources distribute its Biolaxin™ products.

iHerb.com
5012 4th Street
Irwindale, CA 91706
Toll Free: 866-328-1171
www.iherb.com

ProHealth, Inc.
2040 Alameda Padre Serra
Santa Barbara, CA 93103
Toll free: 800-366-6056
www.prohealth.com

FYH (For Your Health/US Biotek Laboratories)
13500 Linden Avenue Ave N.
Seattle, WA 98133
Phone: 206-365-8488
www.foryourhealth.com

Index